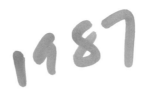

NEUROLARYNGOLOGY
Recent Advances

Edited by

Minoru Hirano, M.D.
Department of Otolaryngology–Head and Neck Surgery
Kurume University Medical School

John A. Kirchner, M.D.
Department of Otolaryngology–Head and Neck Surgery
Yale University School of Medicine

Diane M. Bless, Ph.D.
Department of Communicative Disorders
University of Wisconsin

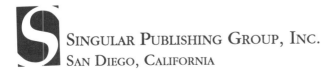

SINGULAR PUBLISHING GROUP, INC.
SAN DIEGO, CALIFORNIA

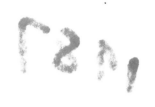

SINGULAR PUBLISHING GROUP, INC.
4284 41ST STREET
SAN DIEGO, CALIFORNIA 92105

Library of Congress Cataloging in Publication Data
Main entry under title:

Neurolaryngology: recent advances.

"A College Hill publication."
Based on a conference held May 16-17, 1986 at the Suikoen Hotel in Kurume, Japan to commemorate the 15th anniversay of Minoru Hirano's professorship.
Includes index.
1. Larynx–Congresses. 2.
Larynx–Innervation–Congresses. 3.
Larynx–Diseases–Congresses.
I. Hirano, Minoru, 1932-   . II. Kirchner, John A., 1915-
III. Bless, Diane M., 1942-   . [DNLM: 1. Laryngeal
Nerves–congresses. 2. Larynx–physiology–congresses.
3. Muscles–physiology–congresses.
4. Neurophysiology–congresses.
WV 500 N4943 1986]
QP306.N48 1987   599'.012   87-16874

ISBN 1-879105-19-5

Printed in the United States of America

Contents

PART 3. **NEUROPHYSIOLOGY**

PART 4. **MUSCLE BEHAVIOR**

PART 5. **PATHOLOGY**

Preface

The Department of Otolaryngology–Head and Neck Surgery, Kurume University and its alumni society were kind enough to propose an event to commemorate the 15th anniversary of my professorship. It was a privilege and pleasure for me to take this opportunity to hold a conference on neurolaryngology.

The conference topic—neurolaryngology—was motivated by three factors: (1) the general lack of knowledge that exists in an area that is critical to many disciplines, (2) the focus of research efforts in our department and in other laboratories in Japan, and (3) the fact that reports of Japanese neurolaryngology research have been limited, in past years, almost exclusively to Japan.

The nerves innervating the larynx account for only a small part of the vagus, one of the 12 cranial nerves. Nevertheless, their functions are tremendously important. They participate in such important functions as airway protection, swallowing, respiration, phonation, speech, and singing. Basic and clinical studies of the neuromuscular system of the larynx have constituted the major thrust of our departmental research during the past quarter century.

Basic and clinical research in neurolaryngology has also been extensively conducted by other otolaryngologists–head and neck surgeons in Japan and in other parts of the world. Unfortunately, the impact of the studies conducted by Japanese researchers has been limited, because many of the reports have been published only in Japanese journals. The occasion of the celebration of my 15th anniversary provided a mechanism for dissemination of this information on a broader scale.

The conference was held on May 16–17, 1986 at Suikoen Hotel in Kurume. The major purposes of the conference were to identify the neurolaryngologic research efforts of each invited participant, to exchange knowledge, experience and ideas among the participants, and to share this information with researchers and clinicians in other parts of the world through publication of the conference proceedings.

Although the official language of the conference was Japanese, the proceedings were written in English. Dr. John A. Kirchner, one of the pioneers in neurolaryngology, kindly joined us as a co-editor of the proceedings. He also contributed two valuable chapters. Dr. Diane Bless, a visiting professor at our medical school, also kindly contributed by editing the proceedings. Great thanks are due to these two good friends.

The book consists of a total of 22 chapters, which are divided into five parts. Part 1 includes seven chapters which deal with localization of motoneurons, distribution of sensory fibers, morphology of sensory nerve endings, autonomic innervation, substance P fibers and neuromuscular junctions of the larynx. Part 2 consists of five chapters dealing with laryngeal muscles. In this section histochemical, mechanical, and contraction properties of laryngeal muscles and muscle spindles are discussed. Part 3 consists of five chapters which deal with neurophysiological aspects of the larynx, including laryngeal reflexes, proprioception, laryngeal-respiratory relationships, brainstem response evoked by laryngeal reflex, and laryngeal responses to auditory stimulations. Two papers in Part 4 discuss muscle behavior for articulation and singing. Part 5 is comprised of three papers dealing with neuromuscular pathologies of the larynx. Thus, the five sections of this book cover a wide range of topics in neurolaryngology.

Some readers may question why we employed the term *neurolaryngology*. Conceptually, neurolaryngology is to the larynx what neurootology is to the ear. Although it has not been widely used, the term neurolaryngology is not new. We were unable to determine who coined the word, but were aware that Dr. David Brewer of Syracuse, and others have used the term on many occasions. But regardless of its origin or frequency of use, we believe that neurolaryngology describes an extremely important area of laryngology and neurology. Research in neurolaryngology appears to be in its developing stage and much research is still needed before we can understand the biological and phonatory functions of the larynx. It would give us great pleasure if this publication proved to be a stimulus to new research and to further advances in neurolaryngology.

We thank College-Hill Press for providing us the opportunity to publish these papers. Thanks are due also to the members of the Department of Otolaryngology–Head and Neck Surgery, Kurume University, and its alumni society, for making this wonderful and significant event possible.

With many thanks.

Minoru Hirano, M.D.

Contributors

Minoru Hirano, M.D.
Professor and Chairman,
Department of Otolaryngology–Head and
Neck Surgery,
School of Medicine,
Kurume University,
Kurume, Japan

Hajime Hirose, M.D.
Professor and Chairman,
Research Institute of Logopedics and
Phoniatrics,
Faculty of Medicine,
University of Tokyo,
Tokyo, Japan

Yasuo Hisa, M.D.
Assistant Professor,
Department of Otolaryngology,
Kyoto Prefectural University of Medicine,
Kyoto, Japan

Yutaka Isogai, M.D.
Chief,
Department of Otolaryngology,
Tokyo Electric Power Hospital,
Tokyo, Japan

Yutaka Joshita, M.D.
Department of Neurology,
Jichi Medical School,
Tochigi, Japan

Takashi Kanda, M.D.
Clinical Professor,
Department of Otolaryngology,
Chiba University,
Chiba, Japan

Takeshi Kanaseki, M.D.
Professor and Chairman,
Department of Neuroanatomy,
Faculty of Medicine,
Kyushu University,
Fukuoka, Japan

Toshio Kaneko, M.D.
Professor and Chairman,
Department of Otolaryngology,
Chiba University,
Chiba, Japan

Hiroyuki Kanetaka, M.D.
Department of Otolaryngology,
The University of Tokushima School of
Medicine,
Tokushima, Japan

Yoichi Katto, M.D.
Department of Otolaryngology–Head and
Neck Surgery,
Ehime University,
Ehime, Japan

John A. Kirchner, M.D.
Professor Emeritus,
Department of Surgery,
Section of Otolaryngology,
Yale University School of Medicine,
New Haven, Connecticut

Yasuo Koike, M.D.
Professor and Chairman,
Department of Otolaryngology,
The University of Tokushima School of
Medicine,
Tokushima, Japan

Tadatsugu Maeyama, M.D.
Assistant Professor,
Department of Otolaryngology,
Saga Medical School,
Saga, Japan

Takao Mitsumasu, M.D.
Department of Otolaryngology–Head and
Neck Surgery,
Kurume University,
School of Medicine,
Kurume, Japan

Mitsutada Miyazaki, M.D.
Department of Otolaryngology,
Chiba University,
Chiba, Japan

Masatoshi Morimoto, M.D.
Department of Neuroanatomy,
Faculty of Medicine,
Kyushu University,
Fukuoka, Japan

Hiroshi Nagata, M.D.
Department of Otolaryngology,
Chiba University,
Chiba, Japan

Noriko K. Nishizawa, M.D.
Department of Otolaryngology,
National Rehabilitation Center Hospital,
Tokorozawa, Japan

Minoru Nomoto, M.D.
Department of Otolaryngology,
Chiba University,
Chiba, Japan

Isao Nozoe, M.D.
Department of Otolaryngology–Head and
Neck Surgery,
School of Medicine, Kurume University,
Kurume, Japan

Shinsaku Nunomura, M.D.
Chief,
Division of Otolaryngology,
Mitsubishi Kobe Hospital,
Kobe, Japan

Hiroshi Okamura, M.D.
Associate Professor,
Department of Otolaryngology–Head and
Neck Surgery,
Ehime University,
Ehime, Japan

Sei-ichi Ryu, M.D.
Assistant Professor,
Department of Otorhinolaryngology,
Faculty of Medicine,
Kyushu University,
Fukuoka, Japan

Shigeji Saito, M.D.
Professor and Chairman,
Department of Otolaryngology,
Keio University,
Tokyo, Japan

Fumihiko Sato, M.D.
Clinical Professor,
Department of Otolaryngology,
Kyoto Prefectural University of Medicine,
Kyoto, Japan

Takemoto Shin, M.D.
Professor and Chairman,
Department of Otolaryngology,
Saga Medical School,
Saga, Japan

Masafumi Suzuki, M.D.
Director,
Department of Otolaryngology,
Yokohama Municipal Center Detection
Center,
Yokohama, Japan

Yasumasa Tanaka, M.D.
Department of Otolaryngology–Head and
Neck Surgery,
School of Medicine,
Kurume University,
Kurume, Japan

Jiro Udaka, M.D.
Assistant Professor,
Department of Otolaryngology,
The University of Tokushima School of
Medicine,
Tokushima, Japan

Shigeru Wada, M.D.
Department of Otolaryngology,
Saga Medical School,
Saga, Japan

Shun Watanabe, M.D.
Department of Otolaryngology,
Saga Medical School,
Saga, Japan

Yuji Yaku, M.D.
Chief,
Department of Head and Neck Surgery,
Tochigi Gan Center,
Tochigi, Japan

Yoshikazu Yoshida, M.D.
Guest Professor,
Department of Otolaryngology–Head and
Neck Surgery,
Kurume University,
School of Medicine,
Kurume, Japan

Toshio Yoshihara, M.D.
Department of Otolaryngology,
Chiba University,
Chiba, Japan

PART 1

Neuroanatomy

神経喉頭科学

CHAPTER 1

Central Location of the Laryngeal Efferent Neurons in the Nucleus Ambiguus of Monkeys

Yoshikazu YOSHIDA,
Yasumasa TANAKA,
Takao MITSUMASU,
Minoru HIRANO,
and Takeshi KANASEKI

There have been many morphological studies of the central location of the laryngeal efferent neurons in the brain stem. These neuroanatomical studies have been performed on dogs (Kosaka, 1909; Szentagothai, 1943; Hisa, Sato, Fukui, Ibata, and Mizukoshi, 1984), cats (Szentagothai, 1943; Koyama, 1951; Gacek, 1975; Lobera, Pasaro, Gonzalez-Baron, and Delgado-Garcia, 1981; Miyazaki, 1982; Yoshida, Miyazaki, Hirano, Shin, and Kanaseki, 1982; Pasaro, Lobera, Gonzalez-Baron and Delgado-Garcia, 1983; Davis and Nail, 1984), rabbits (Bunzel-Federn, 1899; Molhant, 1911-1912; Lawn, 1966; Davis and Nail, 1984),

and rats (Lobera et al., 1981). However, little is known about primates. One exception is the study by Furstenberg and Magielski (1955) describing the motor pattern in the nucleus ambiguus of a monkey. They stated that, in a rostrocaudal pattern of innervation in the nucleus ambiguus for the larynx, the cricothyroid was the most rostral of the cells and the adductor muscle group was the most caudal. The abductor cells of origin were found between the level for the cricothyroid muscle and that for the adductor muscle group.

In our previous investigations (Yoshida, Mitsumasu, Miyazaki, Hirano, and Kanaseki, 1984;

2

Yoshida, Mitsumasu, Hirano, and Kanaseki, 1985a) utilizing the horseradish peroxidase (HRP) technique, we have determined the distribution of the motoneurons in the brain stem of monkeys innervating the vagal and the recurrent laryngeal nerves, and the intrinsic laryngeal muscles. We have also performed similar investigations using cats (Miyazaki, 1982; Yoshida et al., 1982; Yoshida, Miyazaki, Hirano, and Kanaseki, 1985b). In monkeys, motoneurons innervating the vagal nerve were located ipsilaterally in the ambigual and retroambigual nuclei and the dorsal motor nucleus of the vagus. The motoneurons supplying the recurrent laryngeal nerve and the intrinsic laryngeal muscles were situated in the ipsilateral nucleus ambiguus.

Recently, we have also determined the localization of the pharyngeal and esophageal motoneurons located in the nucleus ambiguus. This paper will describe our most recent research on monkeys regarding the central location of the intrinsic laryngeal motoneurons and their relationship with other motoneurons situated in the nucleus ambiguus. It will also relate, by way of discussion, the distribution of labeled cells in the monkey and the cat.

MATERIALS AND METHODS

Forty-two monkeys (*Macaca fuscata*) weighing 2 to 4.5 kg were used in this experiment. We investigated the intrinsic laryngeal muscles: the cricothyroid muscle (CT), the posterior cricoarytenoid muscle (PCA), the thyroarytenoid muscle (TA), the lateral cricoarytenoid muscle (LCA), and the interarytenoid muscle (IA); the pharyngeal constrictor muscles: the cephalopharyngeal muscle (CeP), the hypopharyngeal muscle (HP), the thyropharyngeal muscle (TP), and the cricopharyngeal muscle (CP); the cervical esophageal muscle (CE); the soft palate; the stylopharyngeal muscle (STP); the recurrent laryngeal nerve (RLN) and the nodose ganglion (NG) (Table 1-1). In order to determine the distribution of the vagal motoneurons in the brain stem, we injected HRP solution into the nodose ganglion.

Intramuscular ketamine (10 to 20 mg/kg) was used as general anesthesia. A 30 percent HRP (Toyobo Grade I-C) solution was injected into the exposed muscle belly, ganglion, or nerve, under an operating microscope. Twenty-four to 72 hr after injection, the animals were sacrificed for the purpose of determining the location of motoneurons. Details pertaining to the procedures of HRP injection, perfusing, tissue fixations, section cutting, and mounting have been described in articles in the *Brain Research Bulletin* (Furstenberg and Magielski, 1955) of 1984 and the *Acta Otolaryngol (Stockh)* (Yoshida et al., 1984, 1985a). The sections were examined by bright- or dark-field microscopy.

RESULTS

A summary of the results after injections is shown in Table 1-2. In the present paper, the term "nucleus ambiguus" includes the retrofacial nucleus.

TABLE 1-1.
Subjects for an HRP Study

Subjects			injected	injected(μ)	Location HRP	Volume HRP
Muscle	Vagus nerve	Intrinsic laryngeal muscles	Cricothyroid muscle (CT)			
			Posterior cricoarytenoid muscle (PCA)		Muscle belly	1-3
			Thyroarytenoid muscle (TA)			
			Lateral cricoarytenoid muscle (LCA)			
			Interarytenoid muscle (1A)			
		Pharyngeal constrictor muscles	Cephalopharyngeal muscle (CeP)		Rostral portion of passavant ridge	2-4
			Hypopharyngeal muscle (HP)			
			Thyropharyngeal muscle (TP)		Muscle belly	2-4
			Cricopharyngeal muscle (CP)			
		Esophageal muscle	Cervical esophagus muscle (CE)		Level of thyroid gland	2-4
		Soft palate	Soft palate		Soft palate	1-2
	Glosso pharyngeal nerve	Pharyngeal	Stylopharyngeal muscle (STP)		Muscle belly	1-3
Nerve			Recurrent laryngeal nerve (RLN)		Level of middle portion of thyroid gland	3
			Nodose ganglion (NG)		Ganglion	8-10

Intrinsic Laryngeal Muscles

After injection of HRP into each intrinsic laryngeal muscle, almost all labeled neurons were identified ipsilaterally in the nucleus ambiguus, although a few labeled neurons were also observed in the reticular formation. The motoneurons of the CT were observed in the rostral part of the nucleus ambiguus, whereas those of the other intrinsic laryngeal muscles were recognized in the caudal half.

Cricothyroid Muscle

The labeled cell column for the CT extended from a level near the rostral end of the inferior olivary nucleus (or a level caudal to the facial nucleus) to a level caudal to its middle portion. Labeled neurons of the CT were scattered around the outer area of the compact cell group that has been traditionally identified as the nucleus ambiguus by Nissl staining (Figure 1-1). This distinctive finding was seen at the middle

TABLE 1-2.
Summary of Results

Muscle HRP injected			Labeled cell bodies with HRP			
			Cell column		Arrangement in the nucleus	
Group	Muscle	Side	Rostral end	Caudal end		
Intrinsic laryngeal muscles	CT	Ipsilat.	Caudal to rostral end of IO	Caudal to middle of IO	Scattered, annular fashion	Around compact cell group
	PCA TA		Rostral to the middle of IO	Caudal end of IO	Slightly scattered Aggregated	Medial part Lateral part
	LCA IA		Caudal to rostral end of IO		Sparse	Between PCA and TA motoneurons
Pharyngeal constrictor muscles	CeP HP	Ipsilat.	Caudal end of facial nucleus	Caudal part of rostral half of IO	Compact	Dorsomedial part, compact cell group
	TP CP		Caudal to rostral end of IO		Aggregated	Dorsomedial and ventrolateral, large part of nucleus
Cervical esophageal muscle	CE	Ipsilat.	Rostral to rostral end of IO	Caudal to middle of rostral half of IO	Lightly compact	Small ventrolateral part
Soft palate		Ipsilat.	Middle of rostral half of IO	Middle of IO	Scattered	Ventral part
Pharyngeal muscle	STP	Ipsilat.	Caudal part of facial nucleus	Caudal to rostral end of IO	Scattered	Dorsal part of facial nucleus

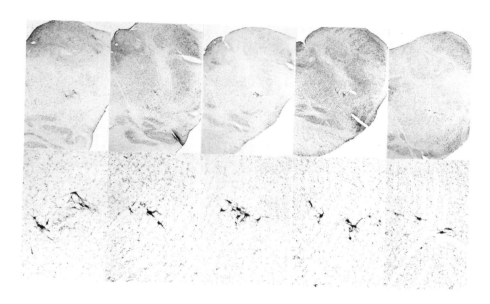

Figure 1-1. *Bright-field photomicrographs of transverse sections of the lower brain stem of monkeys demonstrating the localization of HRP positive cells supplying the cricothyroid muscle (CT), the posterior cricoarytenoid muscle (PCA), the thyroarytenoid muscle (TA), the lateral cricoarytenoid muscle (LCA), and the interarytenoid muscle (IA). Upper line, ×3.2; lower line, ×16.*

level of the CT cell column.

Posterior Cricoarytenoid Muscle

The labeled cell column of the PCA was distributed from a level rostral to the middle of the inferior olivary nucleus (or the most caudal level of the CT cell column) to a level rostral to the caudal end of the inferior olivary nucleus. The levels of each labeled cell column: PCA, TA, LCA, and IA, differed slightly from each other and became more caudal, respectively. However, neither the exact levels of the rostral end of the TA, LCA, and IA labeled cell columns nor the caudal end of the TA and LCA labeled cell columns could

be identified. Labeled cells for the PCA were scattered slightly in the medial part of the nucleus ambiguus (Figure 1-1). A few labeled neurons were also observed dorsomedially in the reticular formation (not including the nucleus ambiguus).

Thyroarytenoid Muscle

The labeled cells for the TA were aggregated in the lateral part of the nucleus ambiguus (Figure 1-1).

Lateral Cricoarytenoid Muscle

The labeled cells for the LCA were sparsely located, between PCA and TA motoneurons, in the middle part of the nucleus ambiguus (Figure 1-1).

Interarytenoid Muscle

IA motoneurons were also sparsely located, between PCA and TA neurons, in the middle part of the nucleus (Figure 1-1). Within this middle part of the nucleus, the LCA motoneurons were identified in the lateral part, whereas the IA neurons were recognized medially. It was observed that the labeled cells of the IA overlapped partially with the TA, LCA, and PCA motoneurons. The caudal end of the IA motoneurons was seen at the caudal end of the inferior olivary nucleus.

Pharyngeal Constrictor Muscles

Following HRP injection into each pharyngeal constrictor muscle, the labeled cell bodies were observed exclusively in the rostral part of the ipsilateral nucleus ambiguus.

Cephalopharyngeal and Hypopharyngeal Muscles

The labeled cell columns for the CeP and the HP extended from the level of the caudal end of the facial nucleus to the level rostral to the middle of the inferior olivary nucleus. The motoneurons of the CeP and the HP were compact and were seen dorsomedially in the nucleus ambiguus. They were located in a compact cell group which has been traditionally identified as part of the nucleus ambiguus by Nissl staining (Figure 1-2).

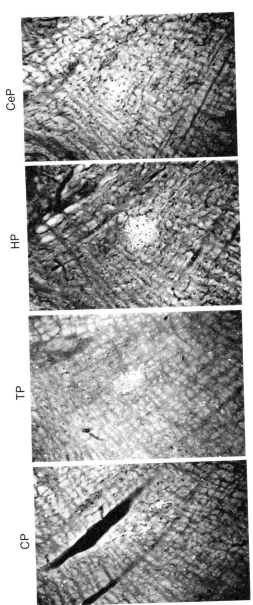

Figure 1-2. *Dark-field photomicrographs of cross sections of the lower brain stem of monkeys showing the location of labeled cells innervating the cephalopharyngeal muscle (CeP), the hypopharyngeal muscle (HP), the thyropharyngeal muscle (TP), and the cricopharyngeal muscle (CP), ×18.*

Thyropharyngeal and Cricopharyngeal Muscles

The labeled cell columns for the TP and the CP extended from a level caudal to the rostral end of the inferior olivary nucleus to a level rostral to the middle of the inferior olivary nucleus. The labeled neurons of the TP and the CP were aggregated in the dorsomedial and ventrolateral parts of the nucleus ambiguus. They occupied a larger portion of the nucleus than the CeP and HP (Figure 1-2). We could not differentiate between the caudal end levels of the pharyngeal constrictor muscle's labeled cell columns.

Cervical Esophageal Muscle

Labeled neurons of the CE were recognized ipsilaterally in the rostral part of the nucleus ambiguus. The labeled cell column for the CE extended from the level caudal to the facial nucleus (or a level rostral to the rostral end of the inferior olivary nucleus) to a level caudal to the middle of the rostral half of the inferior olivary nucleus. The motoneurons of the CE occupied a small ventrolateral part of the nucleus. They appeared slightly compact (Figure 1-3).

The Soft Palate

There are five muscles in the soft palate and the faucium in monkeys (Hartman and Straus, 1971; Swindler and Wood, 1973): the levator muscle of the velum palatinum, the tensor muscle of the velum palatinum, the uvular muscle, the palatoglossal muscle, and the palatopharyngeal muscle. Only the tensor muscle of the

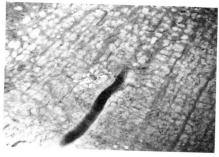

CE

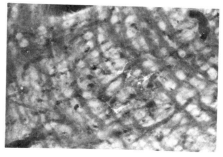

soft palate

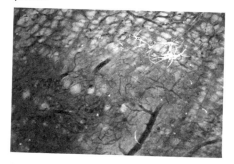

STP

Figure 1-3. Dark-field photomicrographs of transverse sections of the medulla of monkeys demonstrating HRP labeled cervical esophageal (CE), soft palate, and stylopharyngeal (STP) motoneurons, ×50.

velum palatinum is innervated by the third branch of the trigeminal nerve (the mandibular nerve); the remaining muscles are innervated by the pharyngeal plexus. We could not dissect each muscle; therefore, HRP injections were made in the middle portion of one side of the soft palate.

Following injection of HRP into the soft palate, labeled cell bodies were found in the ipsilateral nucleus ambiguus. The labeled cell column of the soft palate was located between the level of the middle of the rostral half of the inferior olivary nucleus and the level of the middle of the inferior olivary nucleus. The soft palate motoneurons were scattered and were located in the ventral part of the nucleus (Figure 1-3).

Stylopharyngeal Muscle

The HRP labeled cells of the STP were only observed in the most rostral part of the nucleus ambiguus ipsilaterally. The labeled cell column for the STP extended from the level of the caudal part of the facial nucleus to a level caudal of the rostral end of the inferior olivary nucleus. STP neurons labeled with HRP were scattered and occupied the area dorsal to facial nucleus in the rostral part of the labeled cell column. They were not within the facial nucleus (Figure 1-3). However, in the caudal part of the STP cell column, the labeled cells were clustered.

Recurrent Laryngeal Nerve

The labeled neurons of the RLN were found in the caudal part of the ipsilateral nucleus ambiguus.

They were distributed between the level just rostral to the middle of the inferior olivary nucleus and the level of the caudal end of the inferior olivary nucleus. The caudal part of the CT labeled cell column and the rostral part of the RLN labeled cell column overlapped. The rostral end of the labeled cell column of the RLN was at the same level as the rostral end of the PCA labeled cell column. The caudal end of the RLN moto-neurons was identical to the level of the caudal end of the IA motoneurons. RLN motoneurons at the level rostral to the obex greatly increased in number, appeared compact in form in the lateral part, and were scattered in the dorsomedial part of the nucleus (Figure 1-4).

Nodose Ganglion

Labeled cells of the vagus nerve at the level of the NG were found ipsilaterally throughout the nucleus ambiguus, including the retrofacial nucleus and the retroambigual nucleus. They led from the level of the caudal part of the facial nucleus (or the level rostral to the inferior olivary nucleus) to C2. When HRP solution was injected into the NG, the neurons in the dorsal motor nucleus of the vagus were also labeled ipsilaterally between the level of the rostral part of the inferior olivary nucleus and C2. The rostral end of the cell column of the nucleus ambiguus was situated at the same level as the rostral end of the STP motoneurons.

The labeled cells of the cell column for the nucleus ambiguus at the level of the rostral third of this

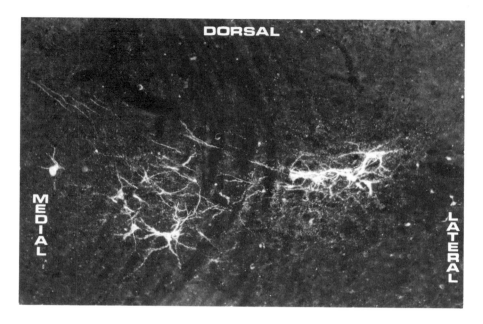

Figure 1-4. *Dark-field photomicrograph of transverse section of the medulla oblongata at the level rostral to the obex. HRP positive recurrent laryngeal motoneurons compact form in ventrolateral part, and scattered in dorsomedial part of nucleus, ×38.*

column increased in number. The labeled cells in the nucleus ambiguus were partially compact, whereas those in the dorsal motor nucleus of the vagus were tightly packed. On the other hand, labeled cells in the retroambigual nucleus were sparse. Several labeled cells were also recognized in the medial reticular formation between the nucleus ambiguus and the dorsal motor nucleus of the vagus along the course of the axons. The arrangements of the motoneurons in the nucleus at each level of A-F, which is depicted in Figure 1-5, is as follows:

A: Level of the Rostral Part of the Nucleus Ambiguus and Level of the Caudal Part of the Facial Nucleus

A few labeled neurons of the nucleus ambiguus were scattered in the outer area dorsal to the facial nucleus, but none were recognized within the facial nucleus (Figure 1-5A).

B and C: Levels of the Rostral Portion of the Inferior Olivary Nucleus

The labeled motoneurons of the nucleus ambiguus were compact and were divided into two groups; the dorsomedial and ventrolateral groups. The dorsomedial group has been traditionally identified as the nucleus ambiguus by Nissl staining. The number of labeled cells in the nucleus ambiguus increased at these levels. The labeled cells of the dorsal motor

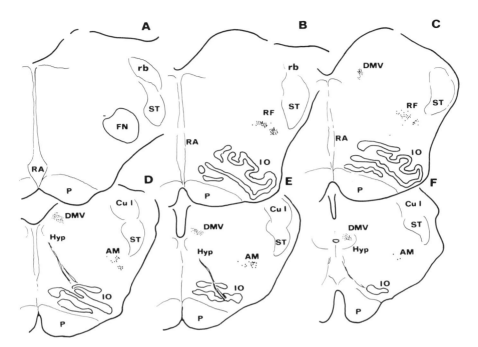

Figure 1-5. *Projection drawings of the labeled neuron distribution in A-F from rostral to caudal levels following HRP injection into the right nodose ganglion of the vagal nerve. A: at the level of the caudal part of the facial nucleus. B and C: at the level of the rostral part of the inferior olivary nucleus. D: at the level of the middle of the inferior olivary nucleus. E: at the level of the rostral portion of the obex. F: at the level of the caudal end of the inferior olivary nucleus. RA, nucleus raphe; P, pyramidal tract; FN, facial nucleus; rb, restiform body; ST, spinal trigeminal tract; IO, inferior olivary nucleus; RF, nucleus retrofacialis; DMV, dorsal motor nucleus of vagus; AM, nucleus ambiguus; Hyp, hypoglossal nucleus and fibers; Cul, nucleus cuneatus lateralis (by Yoshida, Y. et al.,* **Brain Ressearch Bulletin**, *1984).*

nucleus of the vagus showed an aggregated cluster in the nucleus at the level of C (Figures 1-5B, 1-5C).

D: Level of the Middle Section of the Inferior Olivary Nucleus

The motoneurons of the nucleus ambiguus were scattered throughout the nucleus and decreased in number. The cells of the dorsal motor nucleus of the vagus at this level increased in number and

were situated near the fourth ventricle (Figure 1-5D).

E: Level of the Rostral Portion of the Obex

The labeled neurons of the nucleus ambiguus were scattered mediolaterally (Figure 1-5E).

F: Level of the Caudal End of the Inferior Olivary Nucleus

The HRP labeled cells of the

nucleus ambiguus were sparse but located throughout the nucleus. The labeled cell bodies of the dorsal motor nucleus of the vagus were seen near the central canal (Figure 1-5F). The transition from the nucleus ambiguus to the nucleus retroambigualis took place at this level.

DISCUSSION

Distribution of Motoneurons for NG, RLN, and Intrinsic

Laryngeal Muscles in Rostrocaudal Direction

The rostrocaudal extent of the labeled cell columns for the NG, the RLN, and each muscle in monkeys and cats is demonstrated in Figure 1-6. In our previous studies on cats (Yoshida et al., 1985b), following injection of HRP into the NG of the vagal nerve on the ipsilateral side, two labeled cell columns were identified in the ambigual and the retroambigual nuclei (located laterally) and in the

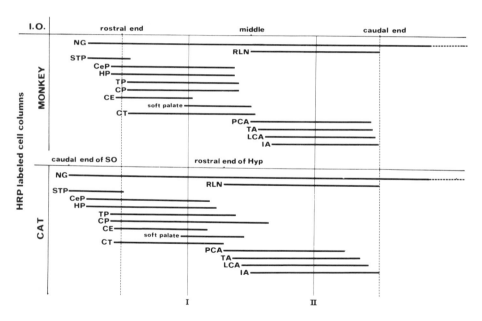

Figure 1-6. *Diagram illustrating the rostrocaudal extent of the labeled cell columns for the nodose ganglion (NG), recurrent laryngeal nerve (RLN), stylopharyngeal muscle (STP), cephalopharyngeal muscle (CeP), hypopharyngeal muscle (HP), thyropharyngeal muscle (TP), cricopharyngeal muscle (CP), cervical esophageal muscle (CE), soft palate, cricothyroid muscle (CT), posterior cricoarytenoid muscle (PCA), thyroarytenoid muscle (TA), lateral cricoarytenoid muscle (LCA), and the interarytenoid muscle (IA), in monkeys and cats. The level in the brain stem is indicated with the cell columns of the inferior olivary nucleus (IO), the superior olivary nucleus (SO), and the hypoglossal nucleus (Hyp).*

dorsal motor nucleus of the vagus (located medially). The former extended between the level of the caudal end of the superior olivary nucleus and C1, and the latter between the level of the rostral end of the inferior olivary nucleus and C2. The extents, in rostrocaudal direction, of these two cell columns in monkeys were basically similar to those of cats. In monkeys, however, the rostral end of the cell column in the ambigual and the retroambigual nuclei were observed at the level of the caudal part of the facial nucleus (or at the level rostral to the rostral end of the inferior olivary nucleus). On the other hand, the caudal end of the nucleus ambiguus was seen at the level of the caudal end of the inferior olivary nucleus and also at the level of the caudal end of the RLN motoneurons.

After HRP injection into the RLN of cats, labeled motoneurons were recognized in the caudal part of the nucleus ambiguus ipsilaterally. They were distributed between the level of the rostral end of the hypoglossal nucleus (or the level of the caudal end of the cell column for the CT) and the level of the caudal end of the inferior olivary nucleus. In monkeys, the rostral end of the labeled cell column of the RLN was at a level rostral to the middle of the inferior olivary nucleus (or the level slightly rostral to the caudal end of the CT motoneurons). This level was the same as the rostral end of the PCA motoneurons. The caudal part of the CT labeled cell column and the rostral part of the RLN labeled cell column overlapped. The caudal end of the labeled cell column of the RLN was at the level of the caudal end of the inferior olivary nucleus in both animals.

The distribution of the CT, the abductor (PCA), and the adductor (TA, LCA, and IA) motoneurons in the rostrocaudal direction was basically the same as reported by almost all previous investigators except Gacek (1975) and Pasaro and colleagues (1983). Gacek (1975) stated that the PCA motoneurons were found in the retrofacial and ambigual nuclei in kittens. According to Pasaro and colleagues (1983), the PCA motoneurons of cats were situated throughout the entire extent of the nucleus ambiguus. In our studies (Yoshida et al., 1982; Yoshida et al., 1985b), labeled neurons of the PCA were not found in such rostral parts. Lobera and colleagues (1981) commented upon Gacek's description, stating that a possible explanation for this difference is the enzyme spread in the kitten to the pharyngeal muscles, causing labeling of the motoneurons located in the rostral part of the nucleus ambiguus. CT motoneurons of both cats and monkeys were situated much more rostrally than the RLN and the remaining intrinsic laryngeal motoneurons. They are close to the pharyngeal motoneurons. As previously described, the reason is understandable as the CT and the pharyngeal constrictor muscles are phylogenetically derived from the fourth branchial arch.

Arrangement of Motoneurons for RLN and Intrinsic Laryngeal Muscles in Transverse Plane

An outline of the arrangement, in transverse plane, of the motoneurons for each muscle of the nucleus ambiguus at two levels in monkeys and cats (I and II in Figure 1-6) is depicted in Figure 1-7.

The RLN motoneurons greatly increased in number at the level rostral to the obex in both cats and monkeys. In cats, they had an aggregated form in the ventromedial and the central parts and a sparse form in the other part of the nucleus ambiguus. By contrast, in monkeys they appeared compact in the lateral part and scattered in the dorsomedial part of the nucleus.

In cats, the CT motoneurons appeared compact in form and were located in the ventral part of the nucleus. By contast, in monkeys they were scattered and were arranged in annular fashion around the outer area of the compact cell group which has been identified as the nucleus ambiguus by Nissl staining.

In cats, the motoneurons of the PCA were aggregated and occupied the middle part of the nucleus, whereas those of the TA were scattered and were seen in the dorsal part of the nucleus. In monkeys, however, the motoneurons for the PCA were scattered and occupied the medial part of the nucleus, whereas those for the TA were aggregated and

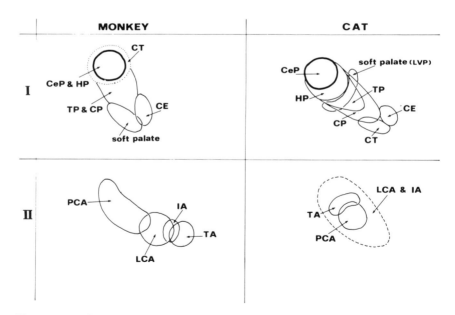

Figure 1-7. *Outline of the somatotopical arrangement of the labeled motoneurons for each muscle in the transverse plane of the nucleus ambiguus at two levels (I and II), which are indicated in Figure 1-6. I: at the level of the middle of the rostral half of the inferior olivary nucleus. II: at the level caudal to the middle of the caudal half of the inferior olivary nucleus. For abbreviations, see Figure 1-6.*

were found in the lateral part of the nucleus. A marked difference in localization of the PCA and the TA motoneurons was observed in both animals. The LCA and IA motoneurons in cats were dispersed widely in the nucleus, whereas in monkeys they were situated in the middle of the nucleus between the PCA and the IA motoneurons. They showed a sparse form in both animals.

On the other hand, according to Davis and Nail (1984), the LCA pool in cats was located in the dorsomedial part of the nucleus. Similar data were obtained from studies on the rabbit. Hisa and colleagues (1984) reported that in dogs, LCA motoneurons were intermingled with TA motoneurons in the dorsal part of the nucleus and the motoneurons of the arytenoid muscle were situated still more dorsally. They also reported that the motoneurons for the adductor muscles (TA, LCA, and arytenoid) were located in the dorsal part of the nucleus, distinctly separate from the motoneurons for the abductor muscle (PCA). This is interesting from the functional point of view of the laryngeal innervation system. Lobera and colleagues (1981) reported that in cats, the laryngeal motoneurons sometimes appear to be clustered in two different groups, one more medial and dorsal than the other, probably indicating a different embryological development. They also proposed that such a specific somadendritic distribution could be related to the dorsal and the ventral location of the expiratory and inspiratory centers, respectively. In the investigation by Pasaro and colleagues (1983) the

dual innervation of laryngeal muscles in cats was demonstrated only for the PCA muscle. In their experiments, HRP injection into the PCA labeled two different motoneuron classes in the nucleus ambiguus with respect to their size. The PCA motoneurons appeared larger in the caudal pole and smaller in the rostral one-third of the nucleus. They also stated, "It may tentatively be said that the smaller neurons supply red tonic fibers and larger neurons supply white phasic fibers." Our results do not agree with this interpretation.

Relationship of Intrinsic Laryngeal Motoneurons with Other Motoneurons Situated in the Nucleus Ambiguus

In our previous investigations (Yoshida et al., 1985b), we defined the myotopical representation of the motoneurons of the nucleus ambiguus in cats. The cell column of the nucleus ambiguus was divided into three parts cytoarchitecturally: the rostral loose, the middle compact, and the caudal loose formations. The rostral loose formation, which was the rostral one-sixth, contained most of the STP motoneurons and part of the CeP and the HP motoneurons. The middle compact formation, which was the next third, was composed of two groups: the large cell group and the compact small cell group. The former, occupying the large region of the nucleus, was located ventrolaterally and supplied the esophageal muscle and the CT. The latter, located in the dorsomedial part, innervated the CeP, the HP and the soft palate. Both innervated the TP and the CP. The caudal loose formation, which was the caudal half, contained the motoneurons for the PCA, the TA, the LCA, and the IA.

In monkeys, the arrangement and density of the labeled cells of the nucleus ambiguus indicated three different types of distribution as in cats: the rostral dispersed, the middle compact, and the caudal loose formations. The rostral dispersed formation contained most of the SPT motoneurons and part of the CeP, the HP, and the CE. The middle compact formation was divided into two groups: the ventrolateral cell group and the dorsomedial cell group. The former, occupying the ventrolateral large region of the nucleus, supplied the motoneurons for the CE and the soft palate. The latter, situated in the dorsomedial small compact region of the nucleus, innervated the CeP and the HP motoneurons. The motoneurons of the TP and the CP were innervated by both groups. The caudal loose formation contained the PCA, the TA, the LCA, and the IA motoneurons. The somatotopical arrangement of the motoneurons of the nucleus ambiguus of monkeys was basically similar to that of cats.

SUMMARY

After injection of HRP into the intrinsic laryngeal muscles, the pharyngeal constrictor muscles, the CE, the soft palate, and the STP of the monkeys, all of the HRP labeled cell bodies were identified in the ipsilateral nucleus ambiguus except for some labeled cells of the PCA. A few labeled neurons of the PCA were found in the reticular formation of the dorsomedial aspect of the nucleus ambiguus. CT motoneurons were scattered around the outer area of a compact cell group of the nucleus ambiguus in the dorsomedial part of the rostral half of the nucleus. PCA, TA, LCA, and IA motoneurons were seen in the caudal half of the nucleus. Within this caudal half of the nucleus, the motoneurons of the PCA were situated in the medial part, those of the TA in the lateral part, and those of the LCA and the IA in the middle part of the nucleus. CeP and HP motoneurons were observed in the rostral half of the nucleus at the dorsomedial part, TP and CP motoneurons at the dorsomedial and ventrolateral parts, CE neurons at the small ventrolateral part, the soft palate motoneurons at the ventral part, and the STP motoneurons at the outer dorsal part of the facial nucleus in the rostral half of the nucleus.

On the basis of our investigations where HRP studies for the NG and the RLN were performed to determine the exact extent of the nucleus ambiguus, we attempted to define the relationship of the intrinsic laryngeal motoneurons with other motoneurons situated in the nucleus ambiguus of monkeys. The cell column of the nucleus ambiguus, which was distributed from the level of the caudal part of the facial nucleus to the level of the caudal end of the inferior olivary nucleus, indicated three different types of arrangement: the rostral dispersed formation, the middle compact formation, and the caudal loose formation. The rostral dispersed formation contained most of the STP motoneurons and part of the CeP, HP, and CE motoneurons.

The middle compact formation was composed of two groups: the ventrolateral cell group and the dorsomedial cell group. The former occupied the ventrolateral large region of the nucleus and supplied the motoneurons for the CE and the soft palate. The latter was located in the dorsomedial small compact region of the nucleus and contained the CeP and the HP motoneurons. Both innervated the TP and the CP motoneurons. The caudal loose formation innervated the PCA, the TA, the LCA, and the IA motoneurons.

The labeled cell distribution in the monkey and the cat was dis-cussed. The extent, in rostro-caudal direction, of labeled cell columns for the intrinsic laryngeal muscles, the pharyngeal con-strictor muscles, the CE, the soft palate, the STP, the RLN, and the vagus nerve in monkeys showed patterns that were basically similar to those of cats. However, the arrangements, in the transverse plane, of motoneurons for the RLN, the CT, the PCA, the TA, the LCA, the IA, and the soft palate indicated a marked difference between monkeys and cats. We believe that the localization of these motoneurons differs between animal species and war-rants further study.

REFERENCES

Bunzel-Federn, E. (1899). Der centrale Ursprung des N. vagus. Monatsschr. f Psychiat Neurol, 5, 1–22.

Davis, P.J., and Nail, B.S. (1984). On the location and size of laryngeal motoneurons in the cat and rabbit. J Comp Neurol, 230, 13–32.

Furstenberg, A.C., and Magielski, J.E. (1955). A motor pattern in the nucleus ambiguus. Its clinical significance. Ann Otol Rhinol Laryngol, 64, 788–793.

Gacek, R.R. (1975). Localization of laryngeal motor neurons in the kitten. Laryngoscope, 85, 1841–1861.

Hartman, C.G., and Straus, W.L., Jr. (1971). The anatomy of the rhesus monkey. New York: Hafner Publishing Co.

Hisa, Y., Sato, F., Fukui, K., Ibata, Y., and Mizukoshi, O. (1984). Nucleus ambiguus motoneurons innervating the canine intrinsic laryngeal muscles by the fluorescent labelling technique. Experimental Neurology, 84, 441–449.

Kosaka, K. (1909). Uber die Vaguskerne des Hundes. Neurol Centralbl, 28, 406–410.

Koyama, H. (1951). The morphological studies on the central innervation of the cat intrinsic laryngeal muscles in the nucleus ambiguus. J Jpn Bronchoesophagol Soc, 2, 31–34.

Lawn, A. M. (1966). The localization, in the nucleus ambiguus of the rabbit, of the cells of origin of motor nerve fibers in the glossopharyngeal nerve and various branches of the vagus nerve by means of retrograde degeneration. J Comp Neurol, 127, 293–306.

Lobera, B., Pasaro, R., Gonzalez-Baron, S., and Delgado-Garcia, J.M. (1981). A morphological study of ambiguus nucleus motoneurons innervating the laryngeal muscles in the rat and cat. Neurosci Lett, 23, 125–130.

Miyazaki, T. (1982). Somatotopical organization of the motoneurons in the nucleus ambiguus of cats—The horseradish peroxidase method—Otologia Fukuoka 28, 649–679.

Molhant, M. (1911-1912). Localizations nuclearies. Le Nevraxe, 12, 277–316.

Pasaro, R., Lobera, B., Gonzalez-Baron, S., and Delgado-Garcia, J.M. (1983). Cytoarchitectonic organization of laryngeal motoneurons within the nucleus ambiguus of the cat. *Experimental Neurology, 82,* 623–634.

Swindler, D.R., and Wood, C.D. (1973). *An atlas of primate gross anatomy, baboon, chimpanzee and man.* Seattle: University of Washington Press.

Szentagothai, J. (1943). Die Lokalisation der Kehlkopfmuskulatur in den Vaguskernen. *Zeitschr F Anat, 112,* 704–710.

Yoshida, Y., Miyazaki, T., Hirano, M., Shin, T., and Kanaseki, T. (1982). Arrangement of motoneurons innervating the intrinsic laryngeal muscles of cats as demonstrated by horseradish peroxidase. *Acta Otolaryng, 94,* 329–334.

Yoshida, Y., Mitsumasu, T., Miyazaki, T., Hirano, M., and Kanaseki, T. (1984). Distribution of motoneurons in the brain stem of monkeys, innervating the larynx. *Brain Res Bull, 13,* 413–419.

Yoshida, Y., Mitsumasu, T., Hirano, M., and Kanaseki, T. (1985a). Somatotopic representation of the laryngeal motoneurons in the medulla of monkeys. *Acta Otolaryngol (Stockh), 100,* 299–303.

Yoshida, Y., Miyazaki, T., Hirano, M., and Kanaseki, T. (1985b). Localization of the laryngeal motoneurons in the brain stem and myotopical representation of the motoneurons in the nucleus ambiguus of cats.—An HRP study—. In I.R. Titze and R.C. Scherer (Eds.), *Vocal fold physiology* (pp. 74–90). Denver: The Denver Center for the Performing Arts.

CHAPTER 2

Localization of the Motoneurons Innervating the Canine Larynx by the Fluorescent Labeling Technique

Yasuo HISA
and Fumihiko SATO

The localization of motor neurons in the nucleus ambiguus that innervate the laryngeal muscles has been investigated using various techniques (Szentagothai, 1943; Furstenberg and Magielski, 1955; Lawn, 1966). The horseradish peroxidase (HRP) method is now the most commonly used tract-tracing technique in the neuronatomical field. This technique has also been used to investigate the location of laryngeal motoneurons (Gacek, 1975; Hinrichsen and Ryan 1981; Lobera, Pasaro, Gonzalez-Baron, and Delgado-Garcia, 1981; Yoshida, Miyazaki, Hirano, Shin, and Kanaseki, 1982). The fluorescent labeling technique, which uses a variety of fluorescent dyes, has recently been reported as an additional tract-tracing technique. (Kuypers, Catsman-Berrevoets, and Padt, 1977; Bentiboglio, Kuypers, Catsmann-Berrevoets, Loewe, and Dann, 1980; Kuypers, 1981). The major advantage of this technique is that it adds the possibility of searching for double-labeled cells. Simultaneous visualization of different cell groups is also made possible for the first time by this technique.

In the present study, we attempted to identify the precise location of the canine motoneurons innervating the intrinsic laryngeal and pharyngeal constrictor muscles, and to detect the existence of double-innervating cells using the fluorescent labeling technique.

MATERIALS AND METHODS

Experiments were performed in 42 2 to 3 month old mongrel dogs (2.5 to 3.5 kg) of both sexes. Under deep anesthesia with ketamine (30 mg/kg, i.m.), fluorescent dyes were injected into the muscles on the right side using a microsyringe. Injection was carefully performed under an operation microscope and the injected points were coated with surgical cement to avoid leakage of tracers. The fluorescent dyes used were 10 percent primuline (Pr) in saline, 3 percent propidium iodide (PI) in saline, 2.5 percent 4',6-diamidino-2-phenylindol-2HCl (DAPI) in distilled water, and 2 percent nuclear yellow (NY) in distilled water. The injected dose was 20 μl each into the cricothyroid muscle (CT) and the thyroarytenoid muscle (TA); and 10 μl each into the posterior cricoarytenoid muscle (PCA), the lateral cricoarytenoid muscle (LCA), the arytenoid muscle (Ar), the hypopharyngeal muscle (HP), the thyropharyngeal muscle (TP), and the cricopharyngeal muscle (CP). The combinations of fluorescent dyes injected into the muscles are shown in Table 2-1 and Table 2-2. Four days after injection, the dogs were anesthetized and perfused with 0.1M phosphate-buffered saline (pH 7.4, at 15°C) followed by a mixture of 4 percent paraformaldehyde and 0.5 percent glutaraldehyde in 0.1M phosphate buffer (pH 7.4, at 15°C). The brain stems were rapidly freed

from the skull and immersed overnight in the same fixative. The tissues were then immersed 1 day in 15 percent sucrose buffered with phosphate (pH 7.4, at 4°C). Frozen transverse serial sections, 40 μm thick, of the lower brain stem were made and washed in phosphate buffer. They were then mounted on chrome-gelatin coated slides in rostrocaudal order and coverslipped with glycerine. They were all examined to detect the neurons labeled with retrogradely transported dyes under an Olympus fluorescence microscope (BH2-RFL) equipped with filter system U and G, providing excitation light of 365 and 546 nm wave length. All labeled neurons were photographed. After fluorescence microscopy, all sections were stained with 0.3 percent carbol-thionin and photographed. The motoneurons labeled with fluorescing tracers on the fluorescence photograph were marked on the corresponding photograph showing carbol-thionin staining to check their location in the nucleus ambiguus.

RESULTS

Intrinsic Laryngeal Muscles

Group A: The cells labeled with PI injected into the CT were located in the rostral part of the nucleus. They extended 1.5 mm caudally from the level immediately caudal to the facial nucleus. The main part of the CT cell column was found at the level of the rostral end of the inferior olive. At this level, the nucleus ambiguus was composed of two divisions: a

Table 2-1.
Injected Intrinsic Laryngeal Muscles of Three Tracers in Four Groups

Group	DAPI	PI	Pr
A	Thyroarytenoid	Cricothyroid	Posterior cricoarytenoid
B	Thyroarytenoid	Lateral cricoarytenoid	Posterior cricoarytenoid
C	Lateral cricoarytenoid	Arytenoid	
D	Arytenoid	Thyroarytenoid	

DAPI: 4', 6 diamidino-2-phenylindol 2HCl
PI : propidium iodide
Pr : primuline

scattered ventral group of larger neurons and a compact dorsal group of smaller ones. The labeled cells were located in the ventral group. The labeled cells with Pr injected into the PCA were found more caudally than the CT cell column. The rostral end of the PCA cell column was located 1.4 mm rostral to the obex where the inferior olive was most prominent. The rostral end of the labeled cell column with DAPI injected into the TA was consistently located just caudal to the rostral end of the PCA cell column. The caudal ends of these two fluorescent cell columns were at nearly the same level, which was 1 mm caudal to the obex. In the transverse plane, the motoneurons in the nucleus were seen to be grouped in two parts at the level where the PCA cell column and the TA cell column were situated. The PCA cells were located in the ventral part and the TA cells in the dorsal part. There was no overlapping of loci of these differently labeled cells.

Group B: The loci of the TA and the PCA cell column were similar to the results in Group A. The LCA cell column labeled with PI was located a little more caudally than the rostral end of the TA cell column. The caudal end of the LCA cell column was also situated a little more caudally than the caudal end of the TA cell column and was near the caudal end of the inferior olive. The LCA cells were intermingled with the TA cells

Table 2-2.
Injected Pharyngeal Constrictor Muscles of Two Tracers in Three Groups

Group	DAPI	NY
E	Hypopharyngeal M.	Thyropharyngeal M.
F	Cricopharyngeal M.	Thyropharyngeal M.
G	Hypopharyngeal M.	Cricopharyngeal M.

DAPI: 4', 6 diamidino-2-phenylindol 2HCl
NY : nuclear yellow

in the dorsal part of the nucleus, whereas the PCA cells were in the rostral part of the nucleus. Double labeled cells were detected only in this group. Those from the TA and the LCA were located at the level just above the obex. These cells were intermingled with the single-labeled TA and LCA cells (Figure 2-1).

Group C: The location of the LCA cell column was similar to that in Group B. The Ar and the LCA cell columns were located at nearly the same level in the nucleus. The Ar cells were located in the most dorsal part of the nucleus in the transverse plane. No double-labeled cells were detected.

Group D: The location of the TA and Ar cells in the nucleus was essentially identical to that in groups A, B, and C. No double-labeled cells were detected.

Pharyngeal Constrictor Muscles

Group E: The HP cell column and the TP cell column were located at nearly the same level in the rostral portion of the nucleus. The rostral ends of these cell columns were located immediately caudal to the facial nucleus and the caudal ends were 2.5 mm rostral to the obex. HP cells and TP cells were intermingled in the dorsal part of the nucleus. No double-labeled cells were detected.

Group F: The rostral end of the CP cell column was located at the same level as that of the TP cell column. However, the caudal end of the CP cell column was more caudal than that of the TP cell column. It was situated 1.8 mm

rostral to the obex. CP cells were mainly located in the ventral part of the nucleus, although TP cells were located in the rostral part. No double-labeled cells were detected.

Group G: The location of the HP cells and the CP cells in the nucleus was essentially identical to that of groups E and F. No double-labeled cells were detected.

These results are summarized in the diagram and the outline drawings on the basis of careful comparisons of many photographic plates (Figure 2-2).

DISCUSSION

In the present study, the application of the fluorescent labeling technique with different tracers for intrinsic laryngeal muscles and pharyngeal constrictor muscles in the same dog made it possible to determine the location of the motoneurons innervating each muscle in the nucleus ambiguus. This characteristic distribution for each intrinsic laryngeal muscle rules out the diffusion of the tracer into neighboring muscles.

The rostrocaudal extension of the motoneurons innervating the laryngeal muscles has been reported in several species: dogs (Szentagothai, 1943), cats (Szentagothai, 1943), rabbits (Lawn, 1966), and monkeys (Furstenberg and Magielski, 1955), using the anterograde or retrograde degeneration technique, and the electrical stimulation technique.

Concerning the intrinsic laryngeal muscles, the retrograde axonal labeling technique has recently been applied to this

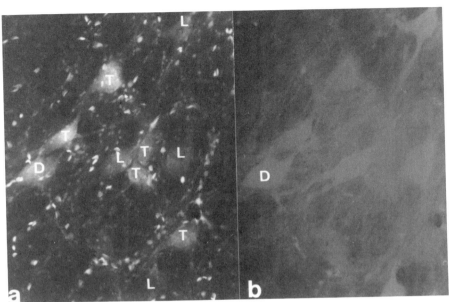

Figure 2-1 A: fluorescent micrograph of the labeled cells in the nucleus ambiguus (filter system U). Blue fluorescent cells labeled with DAPI injected into the thyroarytenoid muscle (T) were intermingled with the dim orange fluorescent cells labeled with propidium iodide (PI) injected into the lateral cricoarytenoid muscle (L) in the dorsal part of the nucleus (× 330). B: fluorescent micrograph of the same section as A (filter system G). Labeled cells with PI were clearly distinguished with brilliant red fluorescence. The doubly labeled cell (D) also had brilliant red fluorescence (× 360).

problem (Gacek, 1975; Hinrichsen and Ryan, 1981; Lobera et al., 1981; Yoshida et al., 1982). Gacek (1975) used the HRP method for the first time to investigate this system in cats. He detected the motoneurons for the CT and the PCA not only in the nucleus ambiguus but also in the retrofacial nucleus, and reported that the CT cell column was situated at nearly the same level for other intrinsic laryngeal muscles in the nucleus ambiguus. However, Yoshida and colleagues (1982), also using the HRP method in cats, reported that only those motoneurons supplying the CT were found in the retrofacial

nucleus and the CT cell column was located in the rostral part, distinct from the other intrinsic laryngeal muscle cell columns in the nucleus ambiguus. The present findings correspond in general with the report of Yoshida and colleagues, although we used dogs as experimental animals. The present findings and previous reports (Szentagothai, 1943; Furstenberg and Magielski, 1955; Lawn, 1966; Yoshida et al., 1982) demonstrating that the CT cell column is located separately for the cell columns for other intrinsic laryngeal muscles in the rostral part of the nucleus ambiguus in several mammalian species is of

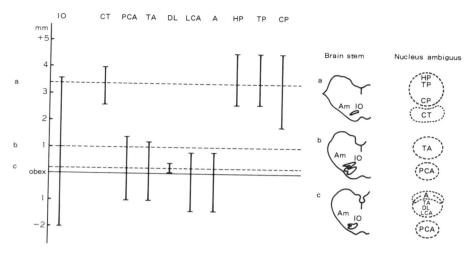

Figure 2-2. The rostrocaudal extension of the labeled cell column in the nucleus ambiguus for each muscle is shown in a diagram. Outline drawings show the transverse sections of the brain stem and the nucleus ambiguus taken through levels A, B, and C in the diagram. A: arytenoid muscle; Am: nucleus ambiguus; CP: cricopharyngeal muscle; CT: cricothyroid muscle; DL: double-labeled cells from the thyroarytenoid and the lateral cricoarytenoid muscles; HP: hypopharyngeal muscle; IO: inferior olive; LCA: lateral cricoarytenoid muscle; PCA: posterior cricoarytenoid muscle; TA: thyroarytenoid muscle; TP: thyropharyngeal muscle.

interest from the phylogenetic point of view. The cricothyroid muscle is known to be derived from the inferior pharyngeal constrictor, a muscle of the fourth arch, whereas all other intrinsic laryngeal muscles are derived from the primordium of the internal constrictor of the sixth arch (Hast, 1972). The present finding that the motoneurons for the pharyngeal constrictor muscles are also located in the rostral part of the muscles, at nearly the same level as the CT cell column, supports this idea. As to the pharyngeal constrictor muscles, Yoshida and colleagues (1981) applied the HRP method for the first time to investigate the location of their motoneurons in the cat. Our results correspond well with their report,

even though the experimental animals are different (cats versus dogs).

The dorsoventral location of the motoneurons for each intrinsic laryngeal muscle and pharyngeal constrictor muscle in the nucleus ambiguus was also defined in this study. Regarding the two cell groups for the TA and the PCA, Yoshida and colleagues (1982) reported that these two cell groups were partially overlapping in the nucleus. However, our study found that these two cell groups never overlapped. One possible explanation for these differences might involve the technique used. The HRP single-labeling technique may not be a reliable method of distinguishing the clear division within the nucleus ambiguus, as the cell column is not continuous and the cells are scattered in the nucleus ambiguus (Taber, 1951). Another possibility is the difference in species, cats versus dogs. The present findings that the motoneurons for the adductor muscles (TA, LCA, and Ar) are located in the dorsal part of the nucleus, distinctly separated from the motoneurons for the abductor muscle (PCA), is interesting from the functional point of view. The application of the fluorescent labeling technique using different dyes also makes possible the simultaneous detection of the dorsoventral location of the motoneurons for each pharyngeal constrictor muscle in the same dog. The finding that there is an obvious difference in the dorsoventral location of the motoneurons for the TP and the CP is interesting, as these two muscles are located close to each other and sometimes look like one muscle.

The most remarkable result in this study using the fluorescent labeling technique is the existence of double-labeled cells. Previous investigators using morphological techniques were unable to detect the existence of motoneurons innervating two different intrinsic laryngeal muscles. Gauthier, Barillot, and Dussardier (1980), by simultaneously recording the discharge of efferent fibers innervating intrinsic laryngeal muscles of the cat, speculated that branches from one motoneuron could innervate both the TA and the LCA. The existence of motoneurons innervating two muscles, the TA and the LCA, was established by this study for the first time. No double-innervating cells for other intrinsic laryngeal muscles or pharyngeal constrictor muscles were found. This finding may be related to the fact that the TA is differentiated from the LCA late in development (Hast, 1972). Functionally, these motoneurons would facilitate the rapid contraction of a part of two synergistic muscles, the TA and the LCA, and contribute to the coordination of vocal fold movements in respiration, deglutition, and phonation.

ACKNOWLEDGMENT

Some parts of this text have been published as original papers (Hisa, Matsui, Sato, Matsuura, Fukui, Tange, and Ibata, 1982; Hisa, Sato, Fukui, Ibata, and Mizuoshi, 1984; Hisa, Sato, Suzuki, Yanohara, Hyuga, and Mizukoshi, 1984).

REFERENCES

Bentiboglio, M., Kuypers, H.G.J.M., Catsmann-Berrevoets, C.E., Loewe, H., and Dann, O. (1980). Two new fluorescent retrograde neuronal tracers which are transported over long distances. *Neurosci Lett, 18*, 25–30.

Furstenberg, A. C., and Magielski, J.E. (1955). A motor patterns in the nucleus ambiguus. *Ann Otol Rhinol Laryngol, 64*, 788–793.

Gacek, R.R. (1975). Localization of laryngeal motor neurons in the kitten. *Laryngoscope, 85*, 1841–1861.

Gauthier, P., Barillot, J.C., and Dussardier, M., (1980). Mise en evidence electrophysiologique de bifrucations d'azone dans le nerf recurrent larynge. *J Physiol (Paris), 76*, 39–48.

Hast, M.H. (1972). Early development of the human laryngeal muscles. *Ann Otol Rhinol Laryngol, 81*, 524–531.

Hinrichsen, C.F.L., and Ryan, A.T. (1981). Localization of laryngeal motoneurons in the rat. *Exp Neurol, 74*, 341–355.

Hisa, Y., Matsui, T., Sato, F., Matsuura, T., Fukui, K., Tange, A., and Ibata, Y. (1982). The localization of the motor neurons innervating the cricothyroid muscle in the adult dog by the fluorescent retrograde axonal labeling technique. *Arch Otorhinolaryngol, 234*, 33–36.

Hisa, Y., Sato, F., Fukui, K., Ibata, Y., and Mizuoshi, O. (1984). Nucleus ambiguus motoneurons innervating the canine intrinsic laryngeal muscles by the fluorescent labeling technique. *Exp Neurol, 84*, 441–449.

Hisa, Y., Sato, F., Suzuki, Y., Yanohara, K., Hyuga, M., and Mizukoshi, O. (1984). The localization of motoneurons innervating the canine pharyngeal constrictor muscles in the posterior larynx by the fluorescent double-labeling technique. *Arch Otolaryngol, 241*, 83–87.

Kuypers, H.G.J.M. (1981). Procedure for retrograde double labeling with fluorescent substances. In L. Heimer and M.J. Robards (Eds.), *Neuroanatomical tract-tracing methods* (pp. 298–303). New York: Plenum.

Kuypers, H.G.J.M., Catsman-Berrevoets, C.E., and Padt, R. D. (1977). Retrograde axonal transport of fluorescent substances in the rat's forebrain. *Neurosci Lett, 6*, 127–135.

Lawn, A.M. (1966). The localization, in the nucleus ambiguus of the rabbit, of the cells of origin of motor nerve fibers in the glossopharyngeal nerve and various branches of the vagus nerve by means of retrograde degeneration. *J Comp Neurol, 127*, 293–306.

Lobera, B., Pasaro, R., Gonzalez-Baron, S., and Delgado-Garcia, J.M. (1981). A morphological study of ambiguus nucleus motoneurons innervating the laryngeal muscles in the rat and cat. *Neurosci Lett, 23*, 125–130.

Szentagothai, J. (1943). Die Lokalisation der Kehlkopfmuskulatur in den Vaguskernen. *Z Anat, 122*, 704–710.

Taber, E. (1951). The cytoarchitecture of the brain stem of the cat. *J Comp Neurol, 116*, 27–69.

Yoshida, T., Miyazaki, T., Hirano, M., Shin, T., Totoki, T., and Kanaseki, T. (1981). Localization of efferent neurons innervating the pharyngeal constrictor muscles and the cervical esophagus muscle in the cat by means of the horseradish peroxidase. *Neurosc Lett, 22*, 91–95.

Yoshida, Y., Miyazaki, T., Hirano, M., Shin, T., and Kanaseki, T. (1982). Arrangement of motoneurons innervating the intrinsic laryngeal muscles of cats as demonstrated by horseradish peroxidase. *Acta Otolaryngol, 94*, 329–334.

CHAPTER 3

Distribution of Sensory Nerve Fibers in the Larynx and Pharynx: An HRP Study in Cats

Yasumasa TANAKA,
Yoshikazu YOSHIDA,
Minoru HIRANO,
Masatoshi MORIMOTO,
and Takeshi KANASEKI

I t is a well known fact that laryngeal sensation is transmitted by the superior laryngeal nerve and part of the inferior laryngeal nerve to the medulla oblongata via the nodose ganglion in which the sensory nerve cells are situated.

Central projections of the afferents of cranial nerves IX and X have been studied in the past, using degeneration (Allen, 1923; Torvik, 1956; Kerr, 1962; Cottle, 1964; Rhoton, O'Leary, and Ferguson, 1966; Culberson and Kimmel, 1972), Golgi (Astrom, 1953), autoradiographic (Beckstead and Nogren, 1979), and horseradish peroxidase (HRP) techniques

(Nicholson and Severin, 1981; Nomura and Mizuno, 1982, 1983).

The peripheral sensory innervation of the larynx and pharynx has been studied by various techniques:

1. The course and distribution of the somatomotor and sensory nerve fibers in mammals were investigated using the silver impregnation technique (Sugano, 1929) and binocular microscopy (Fuse, 1952; Yatake, 1965).

2. The intramucosal and submucosal distribution of nerve fibers and the morphology of their intralaryngeal terminations were studied by means of the silver impregnation technique (Sasaki, 1943, Matsumoto, 1950; Koizumi, 1953; Koenig and von Leden, 1961; Watanabe, 1985).

3. Nerve endings in the human larynx were observed by electron microscopy (Nagai, 1982, Chiba, Watanabe, and Shin, 1985).

4. The sensory innervation of the feline larynx was studied by Nagaishi (1928), and Suzuki and Kirchner (1968).

5. The area innervated by cranial nerve IX was studied clinically and reported by Reichert (1934), Brodal (1947), and Kunc (1964).

However, in the investigations previously mentioned, no distinction was made between the sensory fibers of the IXth and Xth cranial nerves. Therefore, the peripheral course and distribution of the sensory fibers in the larynx and pharynx have thus far remained obscure. Since Kristensson (1971, 1973) first used the HRP technique in tracing motor neurons of the hypoglossal nerve, this technique has been widely used in neuroanatomical studies of various neural systems. In 1982, a new method for tracing peripheral nerve fibers was introduced by Robertson and Aldskogius, who used wheat germ agglutinin-horseradish peroxidase (WGA-HRP) to study cutaneous sensory nerve fibers and their endings; in 1983 the same technique was applied to the study of trigeminal fibers and their sensory terminals (Marfurt and Turner, 1983). The advantage of this technique is that the WGA-HRP conjugate in low concentrations is taken up only by cell bodies and axonal terminals, but is not taken up by undamaged axons (Pugh and Kalia, 1982).

Therefore, in order to delineate the peripheral course and distribution of the laryngeal and the pharyngeal sensory nerves, we injected WGA-HRP into the nodose ganglion of the Xth cranial nerve and the superior and the inferior ganglion (petrosal ganglion) of the IXth cranial nerve. The present report describes our current investigation of the peripheral course and intramucosal distribution of the sensory nerve fibers in the larynx and the pharynx of cats. See Table 3-1 for a list of abbreviations used in this chapter.

MATERIALS AND METHODS

In order to demonstrate the distribution and peripheral course of the sensory nerve fibers of the superior laryngeal nerve (SLN), the inferior laryngeal nerve (ILN) and the glossopharyngeal nerve (IX), the experiments were divided into two groups (Table 3-2):

Group A: The Group A experiments were subdivided into five smaller groups: Groups A-1, 2, 3, 4, and 5. The experiments in Groups A-1 and A-2 were directed toward determining the distribution of sensory nerve fibers within the SLN and ILN. The experiments in Groups A-3, A-4, and A-5 were undertaken to determine the peripheral course of each branch [SLN, ILN, or the external branch of SLN (ext-SLN)]. In this series, 38 cats (500-3200 gm) were used and in all experiments WGA-HRP was injected into the nodose ganglion.

Group B: This group of experiments was designed to delineate

TABLE 3-1.
List of Abbreviations

IXN:	the glossopharyngeal nerve	TC:	the thyroid cartilage
XN:	the vagal nerve	CC:	the cricoid cartilage
12N:	the hypoglossal nerve	AC:	the arytenoid cartilage
NTS:	the nucleus tractus solitarii	HB:	the hyoid bone
ST:	the solitary tract	TA:	the thyroarytenoid muscle
5ST:	the spinal trigeminal tract	LCA:	the lateral cricoarytenoid muscle
CUR:	the cuneate nucleus (rostral division)	PCA:	the posterior cricoarytenoid muscle
IO:	the nucleus of the inferior olive	IA:	the interarytenoid muscle
SLN:	the superior laryngeal nerve	CT:	the cricoarytenoid muscle
int-SLN:	the internal branch of SLN	TF:	the thyroid foramen
ext-SLN:	the external branch of SLN	CF:	the cricoid foramen
ILN:	the inferior laryngeal nerve	PT:	the palatine tonsil
ant.b.:	the anterior branch of int-SLN	SP:	the soft palate
mid.b.:	the middle branch of int-SLN	NP:	the nasopharynx
post.b.:	the posterior branch of int-SLN	OP:	the oropharynx
r.perf.:	the ramus perforans of the posterior branch of ILN	VE:	the vallecula epiglottica
l.t.b.:	the lingual and tonsillar branch of IX N	SG:	the superior ganglion
EC:	the epiglottal cartilage	IG:	the inferior ganglion

the boundary within the hypopharynx between the area innervated by the laryngeal nerve and that innervated by the glossopharyngeal nerve. In this group 18 cats were used and WGA-HRP was injected into the SG and IG of the IXth cranial nerve. Details of the experimental conditions are shown in Table 3-2.

A ten μl microsyringe filled with WGA-HRP conjugate was coupled to a glass micropipette with a tip diameter 40-50 μm. Multiple injections of 2-3 μl for a total of 6 μl of WGA-HRP conjugate solution were made into the nodose ganglion in Group A. In Group B, multiple injections of 0.5-1.0 μl for a total of 3 μl of WGA-HRP conjugate solution were made both into the superior and the inferior ganglion of the IXth nerve. The surgery was performed under an operating microscope.

After surviving 48 hr, the animals were reanesthetized and perfused through the left cardiac ventricle with normal saline followed by 2.5 percent paraformaldehyde and 1.25 percent glutaraldehyde in 0.1M phosphate buffer at pH 7.6, followed by 0.1M phosphate buffer containing 5 percent sucrose. Following perfusion, the brain stem was dissected free and placed in cold 0.1M phosphate buffer with 30 percent sucrose. The tongue, the pharynx, and the larynx were lumped together and divided into three blocks. Each block was trimmed and decalcified with 5 percent ethylene-tetra-acetic-acid (pH 7.2) for 4-7 days. Serial 50 μm transverse frozen sections through the medulla were made in all cases. Serial 50 μm transverse sections of the larynx were made in half of each experimental group (A-1 to A-5); in the other half, serial 50 μm frontal sections were made. Serial 50 μm transverse sections of the pharynx were made in all cases.

TABLE 3-2.
Experiments in six groups demonstrating distribution of sensory nerve fibers using the WGA-HRP technique in cats.

Group of Investigations		Injection Site	Observation	Condition of experiments			Number of Animals
				int-SLN	ext-SLN	ILN	
A	1	Nodose Ganglion	Innervation of SLN and ILN	intact			8
	2		Possible innervation of branches other than SLN and ILN	cut			4
	3		Innervation of SLN	intact		cut	14
	4		Innervation of ILN	cut		intact	8
	5		Innervation of ext-SLN	cut	intact	cut	4
B		Superior Ganglion & Inferior Ganglion	Innervation of glossopharyngeal n.	cut			18

All sections were then treated for HRP activity with tetramethyl benzidine (TMB) in the manner described by Mesulam (1978), and mounted on chrome-alum-gelatin-coated slides. Sections of the medulla were counterstained with neutral red for better orientation of the neural structures. Counter-staining was not used in the laryngeal and pharyngeal sections because it tends to obscure the labeled neural structures in the peripheral organ. All sections were examined by darkfield and light illumination microscopy.

RESULTS

Medulla Oblongata

Following WGA-HRP injection into the nodose ganglion, a large number of labeled vagal nerve terminations were found confined within the nucleus tractus solitarii of the medulla, but none were found in the nucleus ambiguus or the dorsal motor nucleus of the vagus (Figure 3-1).

Similarly, after WGA-HRP was injected into the SG and IG of the IXth cranial nerve, many labeled

glossopharyngeal nerve terminations were found in the nucleus
tractus solitarii, the spinal
trigeminal nucleus, and the medial
cuneate nucleus, but none in the
nucleus ambiguus, the dorsal
motor nucleus of the vagus, or the
inferior salivatory nucleus (Figure
3-2). This indicates that the uptake
of WGA-HRP was limited to cell
bodies of the sensory neurons. In
other words, the labeled
peripheral fibers in these experiments were sensory nerve fibers.

Peripheral Course

The Superior Laryngeal Nerve (SLN)

The labeled SLN fibers
penetrated the thyroid foramen
(Figures 3-4K, 3-5E, 3-7A), traveled
upward and divided into anterior,
middle, and posterior branches
(Figures 3-4G, I, K, 3-5E, G).

1. The anterior branch traveled
ventrorostrally in the direction of
the laryngeal aspect of the epiglottis (Figures 3-4F, G, 3-7C) and a
small anterior part of the aryepiglottic fold.
2. The middle branch traveled
rostromedially and divided into
two groups. One group branched
into many fibers and traveled
toward the aryepiglottic fold, the
rostral aspect of the vocal fold, and
the posterolateral aspect of the
arytenoid eminence (Figures
3-4G,H,I,J, 3-5C, D,E). The second
group penetrated the cricoid
foramen along with the posterior
branches of the int-SLN and ILN
(Figures 3-4J, 3-7B).

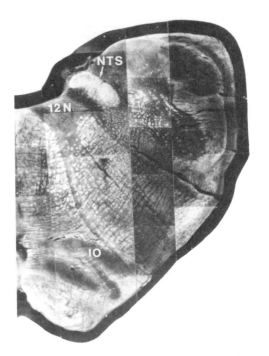

Figure 3-1. *Photomicrograph of HRP labeling of the medulla at levels of the area postrema after WGA-HRP injection into the nodose ganglion. A large number of labeled terminations were recognized in the nucleus tractus solitarii, but no labeled cell bodies were found in the nucleus ambiguus and the dorsal motor nucleus of the vagus. × 12.5.*

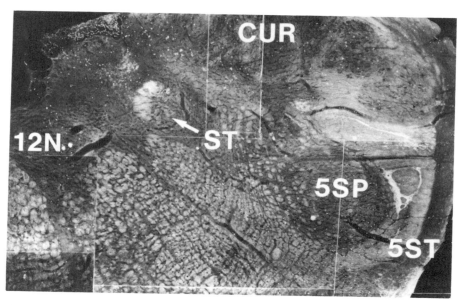

Figure 3-2. *Photomicrograph of HRP labeling of the medulla at levels of the area postrema. Labeled terminations were recognized in the nucleus tractus solitarii, the nucleus tractus spinalis, n. trigemini, and the medial cuneate nucleus, but no labeled cell bodies were found in the nucleus ambiguus, the dorsal motor nucleus of the vagus or reticular formation. ×30.*

3. The posterior branch traveled dorsocaudally and divided into four groups.

The first group of fibers traveled dorsomedially and penetrated the cricoid foramen (CF). This foramen is located near the center of the cricoid lamina near the junction between the rostral one-sixth and the caudal five-sixths of the cartilage. The posterior branch of the ILN and the middle branch of the int-SLN also enter through this foramen (Figures 3-4J,K, 3-7B).

The second group of fibers branched extensively and traveled anteriorly toward the mucous membrane covering the posterior cricoarytenoid muscle (PCA), and toward the lateral and posterior walls of the hypopharynx (Figures 3-4J, K,L, 3-5A,B,C).

The third group of fibers traveled ventrocaudally between the thyroarytenoid (TA) and lateral cricoarytenoid (LCA) muscles, along with the fibers in the posterior branch of the ILN, and traveled toward the subglottis (Figure 3-5G).

The fourth group of fibers traveled caudally and connected with the posterior branch fibers of the ILN and formed Galen's anastomosis.

The Inferior Laryngeal Nerve (ILN)

The labeled sensory nerve fibers of the ILN traveled rostrally in the submucosal layer of the anterior aspect of the hypopharynx, ran between the thyroid cartilage (TC) and the PCA muscle (Figures 3-4J,K,L, 3-5A,B,C,D), and divided into two branches.

One traveled rostrally and formed Galen's anastomosis. The other ran ventrorostrally to pass between the LCA and the TA together with the third group of the posterior branch of the int-SLN. In this paper this fiber bundle will be called the ramus perforans (Figures 3-4J, 3-5G).

The Glossopharyngeal Nerve (IX N)

The labeled sensory nerve fibers of the lingual and tonsillar branch penetrated the pharyngeal muscles surrounding the pharynx at the level of the caudal pole of the palatine tonsil and divided into four rami (Figure 3-4A).

1. The first ramus ran rostrally in the radix of the tongue with many small branches (Figure 3-4A).

2. The second ramus traveled rostrally around the palatine tonsil and gradually branched into separate fibers until it reached the soft palate (Figure 3-4A).

3. The third ramus traveled ventrocaudally toward the vallecula epiglottica and the lingual aspect of the epiglottis (Figure 3-4B,C,D).

4. The fourth ramus ran dorsolaterally and caudally and gradually branched into separate fibers until reaching the lateral and dorsal walls of the hypopharynx (Figure 3-4A,B,C,D,E,F).

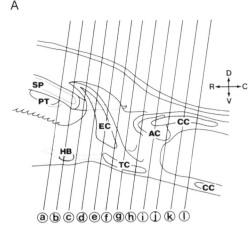

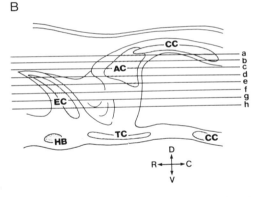

Figure 3-3. *A: Figure showing the location of the cutting plane indicated in Figure 3-4. B: Figure showing the location of the cutting plane indicated in Figure 3-5.*

Distribution

The Superior Laryngeal Nerve (SLN)

1. The anterior branch of the int-SLN innervated the laryngeal aspect of the epiglottis (Figures 3-4G, 3-7C) and a small part of the aryepiglottic fold ipsilaterally.

2. The middle branch of the int-SLN innervated two areas. One group innervated most parts of the aryepiglottic fold (Figures 3-4G,H, 3-7D), the posterolateral aspects of the arytenoid eminence (Figure 3-4H) and the laryngeal vestibulum ipsilaterally. The other group, penetrating the CF, innervated the inner aspect of the arytenoid cartilage and the posterior wall of the glottis. Although the innervation crossed the midline, ipsilateral predominance was present (Figures 3-4I,J,K, 3-5A, B,C).

3. The posterior branch of the int-SLN innervated four areas.

The first group of fibers joined the middle branches of the int-SLN and the ILN, and supplied the same areas as those innervated by the second group of the middle branch of the int-SLN (Figures 3-4I,J,K, 3-5A,B,C).

The second group innervated the mucous membrane covering the PCA in the hypopharynx, and the lateral and posterior walls of the hypopharynx ipsilaterally. The sensory nerve fibers of this group supplied an area extending from the middle of the aryepiglottic fold to the level of the caudal end of the piriform sinus (Figure 3-4G,H,I,J, K,L).

The third group supplied the caudal aspect of the vocal fold

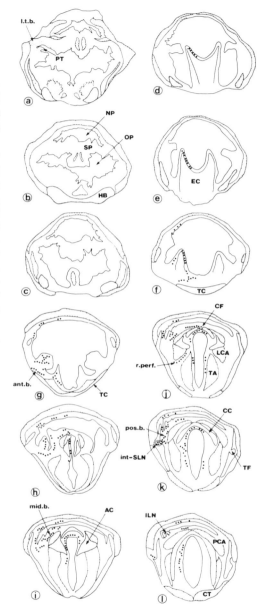

Figure 3-4. *Schematic drawings outlining peripheral course and intra-mucosal distribution of HRP labeled sensory nerve fibers of int-SLN (filled circles), ILN (filled triangles), and IXth cranial nerve (open triangles) in transverse section of the pharynx and larynx. Consecutive planes indicated by circled letter.*

and the subglottis (Figure 3-5F,G,H).

The fourth group formed Galen's anastomosis with the posterior branch of ILN.

The Inferior Laryngeal Nerve (ILN)

Except for the branch forming Galen's anastomosis, the sensory nerve fibers of the ILN innervated the caudal aspect of the vocal fold and the subglottis bilaterally, but with ipsilateral predominance (Figures 3-4J,K,L, 3-5C,D,F,G,H).

The Glossopharyngeal Nerve (IX N)

The labeled sensory nerve fibers of the IXth cranial nerve were recognized ipsilaterally in the epipharynx, the caudal half of the soft palate (both oral and nasopharyngeal aspects) (Figures 3-4A,B,C,D, 3-8C), the caudal third of the tongue (Figures 3-4A,C, 3-8B), the vallecula epiglottica (Figures 3-4C,D, 3-8D), the lingual aspect of the epiglottis (Figure 3-4D), and the pharyngeal wall (Figure 3-4A,B,C,D,E,F).

The first ramus innervated the caudal one-third of the tongue ipsilaterally, except for the vallecula epiglottica and the vallate papillae (Figure 3-8B). The second ramus innervated the palatine tonsil (Figures 3-4A, 3-8A) and the caudal half of the soft palate ipsilaterally (both oral and nasopharyngeal aspects) (Figures 3-4A,B,C,D, 3-8C). The third ramus supplied a part of the radix of the tongue, the vallecula epiglottica (Figures 3-4C,D, 3-8D) and the lingual aspect of the epiglottis (Figure 3-4D). The fourth ramus

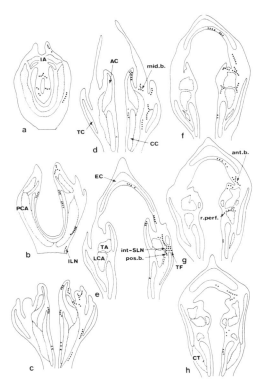

Figure 3-5. *Schematic drawings outlining peripheral course and intramucosal distribution of HRP labeled sensory nerve fibers of int-SLN (filled circles) and ILN (filled triangles) investigated in horizontal sections of the larynx. Consecutive planes indicated by letter.*

innervated the lateral and the posterior walls of the hypopharynx rostral to the level corresponding to the level of the middle level of the aryepiglottic fold (Figure 3-4A,B,C,D,E,F).

In this study, no labeled sensory nerve fibers of the SLN or the ILN were found in the mucosa of the vallecula epiglottica. In the mucosa of the lingual aspect of the epiglottis we found that the labeled sensory fibers were derived from the IXth cranial nerve, whereas in the mucosa of the laryngeal aspect of the epiglottis we found that the labeled sensory nerve fibers were derived from the Xth.

In the mucous membrane of the lateral and posterior walls of the hypopharynx we found labeled fibers of the IXth nerve rostral to the mid-level of the aryepiglottic fold; we also found labeled fibers of the Xth nerve caudal to this section (Figures 3-4F, 3-6A, 3-6B). At this level there may be a double innervation by the IXth and Xth nerves. However, we were unable to identify any areas of double innervation in the hypopharynx.

A summary of the findings of this study is found in Table 3-3.

DISCUSSION

According to previous studies using degeneration (Allen, 1923; Torvik, 1956; Kerr, 1962; Cottle, 1964; Rhoton et al., 1966; Culberson and Kimmel, 1972), Golgi (Astrom, 1953), autoradiographic (Beckstead and Norgren, 1979), and HRP methods (Nicholson and Severin, 1981; Nomura and Mizuno, 1982, 1983), the medullary projection of the afferents of the Xth or IXth cranial nerve complex is in the nucleus

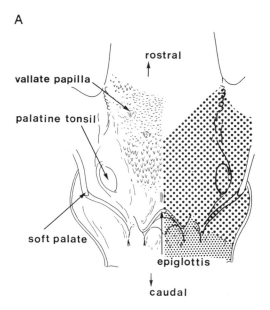

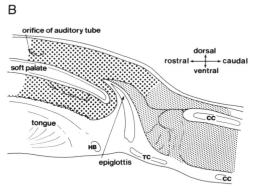

Figure 3-6. *Figures showing the distribution of IXth cranial nerve (large black dots) and the distribution of Xth cranial nerve (small black dots). A: dorsal aspect of the caudal third of the tongue and larynx. B: sagittal section (medial aspect) of the pharynx and larynx.*

TABLE 3-3.
Summary of results in which distribution of laryngeal and glossopharyngeal sensory nerve fibers in cats was investigated by the WGA-HRP technique.

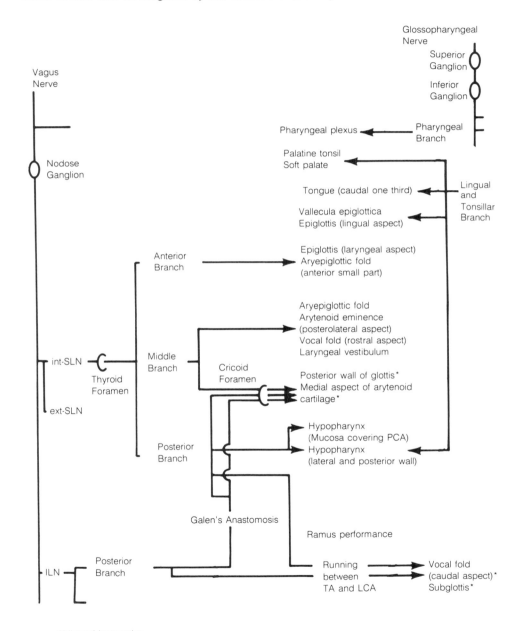

*bilateral innervation.

tractus solitarii and the nucleus tractus spinalis n. trigemini. In addition, Nomura and Mizuno (1983) stated that HRP injected into the SLN resulted in labeling of axon terminals in the solitary nucleus, the principal sensory and spinal trigeminal nuclei, the medial cuneate nucleus, and the dorsal horn of the C1 and C2 cord segment. Application of HRP to the cervical trunk of the IXth nerve produced labeling of axon terminals in the solitary nucleus, the spinal trigeminal nucleus, and the medial cuneate nucleus. In this study, the results of injecting WGA-HRP into the superior and the inferior ganglion of the IXth nerve were in accordance with the latter results, whereas, following WGA-HRP injection into the nodose ganglion, labeled terminations were found only in the nucleus tractus solitarii. In the present study, it was only the afferent components of the IXth and the Xth cranial nerves that were labeled. The nuclei of neither the motor nor the visceral motor neurons were labeled. This demonstrates that the tracer is not taken up by the passing fibers. Therefore, labeled peripheral nerve fibers in the larynx and pharynx are believed to be only sensory nerve fibers.

The course and distribution of the int-SLN, ext-SLN, and RLN in the larynx were investigated by Sugano in dogs (1929) and Yatake in nine species of mammals (1965). Their results can be summarized as follows: In the dog, the int-SLN is divided into two or three branches: the anterior and posterior branches or the anterior, middle, and posterior branches. The anterior branch or the anterior and middle branches supply the

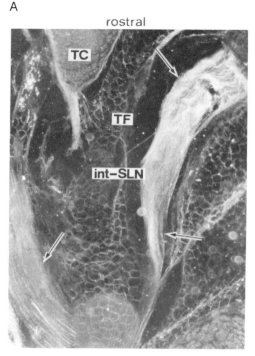

A

rostral

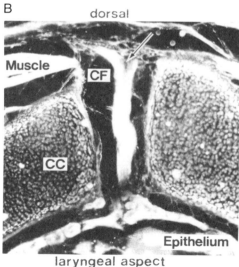

B

dorsal

laryngeal aspect

Figure 3-7. *Photomicrographs displaying four selected sections of the larynx. Arrows indicate labeled sensory fibers. A: horizontal section of the right thyroid foramen. ×40 (darkfield). B: transverse section of the cricoid foramen.*

(continued page 39)

epiglottis. The posterior branch is divided into two groups. One group innervates the posterior part of the larynx to the level of the vocal fold. The other group connects with the posterior branch of the ILN. The posterior branch of the ILN runs upward in the submucosa covering the PCA and forms Galen's anastomosis, uniting with the posterior branch fibers of the int-SLN (Sugano, 1929; Yatake, 1965). In the cat, the int-SLN penetrates the thyroid foramen and is divided into anterior, middle, and posterior branches. The anterior branch innervates both the lingual and laryngeal aspects of the epiglottis. The middle branch supplies the aryepiglottic fold and the laryngeal vestibulum. The posterior branch runs backward and downward below the aryepiglottic fold and, after passing through the submucosa of the processus muscularis of the arytenoid cartilage, reaches the lateral part of the PCA, forming Galen's anastomosis with the posterior branch of the ILN. The course and distribution of the int-SLN in the cat are similar to that in the human. The ILN divides into anterior and posterior branches at the level caudal to the inferior pharyngeal constrictor muscle. The posterior branch of the ILN branches out in the hypopharynx and connects finally with the posterior branch of the int-SLN as Galen's anastomosis (Yatake, 1965). In these reports, minute distributions of nerve fibers and density of nerve fibers and endings in mucosa were not described. Our present results agree, in general, with their descriptions. In the present investigation, however, the distribution of sensory nerve fibers

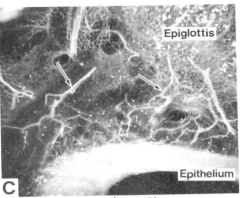

laryngeal aspect

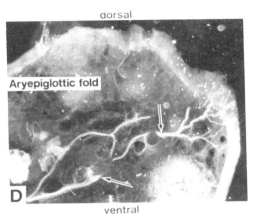

Figure 3-7 (continued).

×40 (darkfield). C: transverse section of right side of the epiglottis. ×40 (darkfield). D: transverse section of the right aryepiglottic fold. ×40 (darkfield).

and the laterality of sensory innervation was clearly detailed.

The submucosal plexus and intramucosal nerve endings of the larynx have been studied in the human (Sasaki, 1943; Matsumoto, 1950; Koenig and von Leden, 1961; Watanabe, 1985) and in dogs (Koizumi, 1953). Sasaki (1943) reported that the submucosal plexus formation and many sensory nerve endings were observed in the laryngeal aspect of the epiglottis in the human larynx. Matsumoto (1950) supported Sasaki's description and stated that the development of the submucosal plexus and intramucosal sensory nerve endings was paralleled in the human larynx. Sensitivity was more acute in the laryngeal vestibulum than in other parts of the larynx. The richest areas of sensory innervation were the laryngeal aspect of the epiglottis, the aryepiglottic fold, and the pars intercartilagina, respectively. In the vocal fold, the density of sensory nerve fibers was heavier in the posterior region than in the anterior (Koizumi, 1953). Koenig and von Leden (1961) stated that the sensory innervation of the mucosa differed widely in the anterior and posterior segments of the vocal fold. They found a definite network of neurofibrils in the posterior third of each vocal fold. By contrast, they could not establish any network of neurofibrils in the mucosa covering the anterior two-thirds of the vocal fold. Furthermore, they encountered a deeply placed network of neurofibrils in the interarytenoid notch and in the laryngeal portion of the hypopharynx. Watanabe (1985) also supported their description.

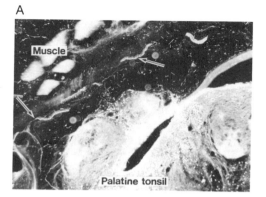

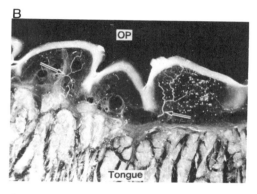

Figure 3-8. *Photomicrographs displaying four selected sections of the pharynx. Arrows indicate labeled sensory fibers. A: transverse section of the right palatine tonsil and its surroundings. ×30 (darkfield). B: transverse section of right side of the mucous membrane of the radix of the tongue. ×30 (darkfield). C: transverse section of right side of the soft palate. ×40 (darkfield). D: transverse section of right side of the vallecula epiglottica. ×192 (darkfield).*

(continued page 41)

Our studies of the development of sensory nerve fibers of the laryngeal mucosa support their conclusions.

Afferent components in the ILN have been reported. Lemere, studying dogs (1932), and Rustad and Morrison (1952) and Williams (1954), studying humans recognized sensory fibers of the ILN. Nomura and Mizuno (1983) identified that following HRP application to the ILN, many terminations appeared in the nucleus tractus solitarii. In this study, following WGA-HRP injection into the nodose ganglion, in the case of group A-1, numerous sensory nerve fibers and terminations were found in the ILN and the nucleus tractus solitarii.

As for the region supplied by the SLN or the ILN, Nagaishi (1983) reported that the SLN innervated the supraglottic region ipsilaterally and its innervation spread as far as the upper region of the trachea. Hirose (1961) observed that it was generally agreed that the sensory nerve fibers of the SLN innervated only the supraglottic region ipsilaterally. In the present study, the int-SLN innervated not only the supraglottic region but also the subglottic region; the former was innervated ipsilaterally, whereas the latter was supplied bilaterally.

The possibility of the ext-SLN containing a large proportion of afferent fibers was suggested in a physiological study of the cat (Suzuki and Kirchner, 1968). Afferent impulses were recorded from filaments of the ext-SLN in response to touch and pressure applied to the mucosa and deep structures of the anterior subglottic midline area of the larynx. This area was roughly diamond-

C

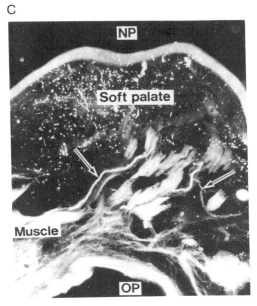

D

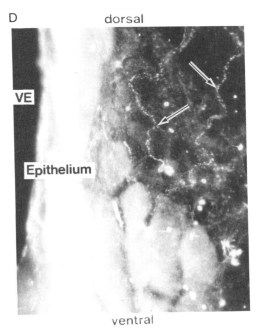

Figure 3-8 (continued).

shaped and extended from the inferior border of the thyroid cartilage above to the superior border of the first tracheal ring below. In the present experiments, in the case of group A-5, no labeled sensory nerve fibers were found in the mucosa of this area.

The cricoid foramen that was situated in the midline of the lamina of the cricoid cartilage near the junction of its rostral and middle thirds acted as a passageway for fibers of the int-SLN with some fibers of the posterior branch of the ILN. In a few cases, not only a single foramen but two or three foramina were observed in the cricoid plate. The nerve fibers penetrating the cricoid foramen crossed the midline, but showed an ipsilateral predominance. It might be surmised that the cricoid foramen plays an important role in bilateral sensation. The cricoid foramen named by the present authors has, to our knowledge, never been described before. We are not prepared to say if this foramen exists in other mammals.

It has long been known that the glossopharyngeal nerve supplies taste and general sensory fibers to the mucous membrane of the pharynx, except for a part of the epipharynx and hypopharynx, and to the mucous membrane of the posterior third of the tongue (including the vallate papillae) . Glossopharyngeal innervation has been studied in considerable detail. Reichert (1934), Brodal (1947), and Kunc (1964) determined the area of IXth nerve innervation by intracranial tractotomy in patients suffering from glossopharyngeal neuralgia. Accord-

ing to Reichert, observations of the effects of intracranial section of the IXth nerve, in which no injury was inflicted on adjacent nerves, particularly the Xth, are uniform as to the existence of permanent unilateral anesthesia of the soft palate, the pharyngeal wall from the eustachian tube to the epiglottis, and the posterior third of the tongue. In the present study, we found that the area of glossopharyngeal innervation extends from the orifice of the auditory tube to the lateral and posterior walls of the hypopharynx at the mid-level of the aryepiglottic fold as measured in a rostrocaudal direction. Our results agree in general with Reichert's description.

The present investigation identified the circumference of the caudal pole of the palatine tonsil as the area of greatest sensory innervation.

In many research reports the innervation of the lingual aspect of the epiglottis was supplied by the int-SLN and the vallecula epiglottica by both the int-SLN and the glossopharyngeal nerve. Tomita (1974) stated that the glossopharyngeal nerve was also distributed to the lingual aspect of the epiglottis and the vallecula epiglottica. He also stated that a branch of the int-SLN supplied a part of the mucosa of the radix of the tongue. In the present study, labeled nerve fibers derived from the IXth nerve were observed in the mucous membrane of the lingual aspect of the epiglottis and the vallecula epiglottica, but labeled nerve fibers derived from the Xth nerve were not observed. It must be remembered that the innervation of these areas differs in cats and in humans. The variation may be due to the point of entry by the int-SLN: in the human the int-SLN penetrates the thyrohyoid membrane, whereas in cats it penetrates the thyroid foramen and enters the larynx at the level of the vocal fold.

The several pharyngeal branches of the IXth cranial nerve joined the vagus and sympathetic fibers at the level of the middle pharyngeal constrictor muscle to form the pharyngeal plexus. This plexus supplies the muscles and mucous membrane of the pharynx. In this study, following WGA-HRP injection into the nodose ganglion, labeled nerve fibers were not observed in the mucous membrane of the lateral or posterior wall of the pharynx rostral to the level of the mid-aryepiglottic fold. After injection of WGA-HRP into the SG and IG of the IXth nerve, numerous labeled nerve fibers of the lingual and tonsillar branch of the IXth nerve appeared in the pharynx. In addition, there were some labeled nerve fibers that did not belong to its four rami. According to Nomura and Mizuno (1983), no afferent components were labeled after application of HRP to the pharyngeal branch of the vagus nerve. Therefore, labeled nerve fibers that did not belong to its four rami were believed to be fibers derived from pharyngeal branches of the IXth cranial nerve.

We believe that the present data on the peripheral sensory innervation of the larynx and pharynx may be useful in understanding physiological mechanisms in the swallowing reflex and in protective reflex glottic closure.

CONCLUSION

Following WGA-HRP injection into the nodose ganglion of cats, the peripheral and intramucosal distributions of sensory nerve fibers in the larynx and hypopharynx were traced. In addition, to clarify the hypopharyngeal boundary between the areas innervated by the laryngeal nerve and the glossopharyngeal nerve, WGA-HRP was injected into the superior and the inferior ganglion of the IXth cranial nerve.

The results were as follows:

1. The int-SLN divided into three branches and innervated ipsilaterally the laryngeal aspect of the epiglottis, the aryepiglottic fold, the arytenoid eminence, the rostral aspect of the vocal fold, the laryngeal vestibulum, the mucosa covering the PCA, and the lateral and posterior mucosa of the hypopharynx between the mid-level of the aryepiglottic fold and the level of the caudal end of the pyriform sinus.

2. The posterior branch of the ILN divided into two branches. One formed Galen's anastomosis together with fibers of the int-SLN. The other was distributed to the caudal aspect of the vocal folds and to the subglottis, together with fibers of the int-SLN.

3. Some of the fibers of the int-SLN united with some of the fibers of the posterior branch of the ILN and penetrated the cricoid foramen to innervate the posterior wall of the glottis and the medial aspect of the arytenoid cartilage bilaterally, with ipsilateral predominance.

4. The lingual and tonsillar branch of the IXth nerve divided into four rami. One of them supplied the vallecula epiglottica and the oral aspect of the epiglottis ipsilaterally. One of the remaining rami innervated the lateral and posterior mucosa of the hypopharynx rostral to the level corresponding to the mid-aryepiglottic fold.

REFERENCES

Allen, W.F. (1923). Origin and distribution of the tractus solitarius in the guinea pig. *J. Comp. Neurol. 35*, 171–311.

Astrom, K.E. (1953). On the central course of afferent fibers in the trigeminal, facial, glossopharyngeal, and vagal nerves and their nuclei in the mouse. *Acta Phisiol Scand, 29,* 209–320.

Beckstead, R.M., and Nogren, R. (1979). An autoradiographic examination of the central distribution of the trigeminal, facial, glossopharyngeal, and vagal nerves in the monkey. *J. Com. Neurol. 184,* 455–472.

Brodal, A.L.F. (1947). Central course of afferent fibers for pain in facial, glossopharyngeal and vagus nerves. *Arch. Neurol & Psychiat 57,* 292–306.

Chiba, T., Watanabe, S., and Shin, T. (1985). Ultrastructure of the glomerular corpuscular nerve endings in the subepithelium of human epiglottis. *Arch. histol. jap. 48,* 213–221.

Cottle, M.K. (1964). Degeneration studies of primary afferents of IXth and Xth cranial nerves in the cat. *J. Comp. Neurol. 122,* 329–345.

Culberson, J.L., Kimmel, D.L. (1972). Central distribution of primary afferent fibers of glossopharyngeal and vagal nerves in opossum didelphisvirginiana. *Brain Res, 44*(2), 325.

Fuse, T. (1952). Anatomical study of the glossopharyngeal nerve and the plexus intercaroticus. [Japanese]. *Acta Anat. Niigata's ensia, 29,* 148–210.

Hirose, H. (1961). Afferent impulses in the recurrent laryngeal nerve in the cat. *Laryngoscope, 71,* 1196–1206.

Kerr, F.W.L. (1962). Facial, vagal and glossopharyngeal nerves in the cat. *Arch. Neurol. 6,* 264–281.

Koenig, W.F., and von Leden, H. (1961). The peripheral nervous system of the human larynx, Part I. The mucous membrane. *Arch. Otolaryngol., 73,* 1–14.

Koizumi, H. (1953). On sensory innervation of larynx in dog. *Tohoku j. Exp. Med. 58,* 199–201.

Kristensson, K., Olsson, Y., and Sjostrand, J. (1971). Axonal uptake and retrograde transport of exogenous proteins in the hypoglossal nerve. *Brain Res. 32,* 399–406.

Kristensson, K., Olsson, Y. (1973). Uptake and retrograde axonal transport of protein tracers in hypoglossal neurons–Fate of tracer and reaction of nerve cell bodies. *Acta Neurop, 23*(1); 43–47.

Kunc, Z. (1964). Treatment of essential neuralgia of the 9th Nerve by selective tractotomy. *J of neurosurgery 23,* 494–500.

Lemere, F. (1932). Innervation of the larynx. I. Innervation of laryngeal muscle. *An J. Anat, 51,* 417–437.

Marfurt, C.F., and Turner, D.F. (1983). Sensory nerve endings in the rat oro-facial region labeled by the anterograde and transganglionic transport of horseradish peroxidase: a new method for tracing peripheral nerve fibers. *Brain Res. 261,* 1–12.

Matsumoto, K. (1950). Innervation, especially the sensory innervation of the laryngeal mucous membrane except the epiglottis. *Tohoku Med. J. 45*, 11–18.

Mesulum, M. M. (1978). Tetramethyl benzidine for horseradish peroxidase neurohistochemistry: a non-carcinogenic blue reaction-product with superior sensitivity for visualizing neural afferents and efferents. *J. Histochem. Cytochem. 26*, 106–117.

Nagai, T. (1982). Encapsulated sensory corpuscle in the mucosa of human vocal cord: An electron microscope study. *Arch. histol. jap. 45*, 145–153.

Nagaishi, C. (1983). Experimental study of vocal cord movement. *Pract. Otol. (Kyoto) 33*, 518–725.

Nicholsen, J.E., and Severin, C.M. (1981). The superior and inferior salivatory nuclei in the rat. *Neurosci Lett*, 21, 149–154.

Nomura, S., and Mizuno, N. (1982). Central distribution of afferent and efferent components of the glossopharyngeal nerve: An HRP study in the cat. *Brain Res. 236*, 1–13.

Nomura, S., and Mizuno, N. (1983). Central distribution of efferent and afferent components of the cervical branches of the vagus nerve, a HRP study in the cat. *Anat. Embryol. 166*, 1–18.

Pugh, W.W., and Kalia, M. (1982). Differential uptake of peroxidase (HRP) and peroxidase-lectin (HRP-WGA) conjugate injected in the nodose ganglion of the cat. *J. Histochem. Cytochem. 30*, 887–894.

Reichert, F.L. (1934). Neuralgias of the glossopharyngeal nerve with particular reference to the sensory, gustatory and secretory functions of the nerve. *Arch. Neurol. & Psychiat. 32*, 1030–1037.

Rhoton, A.L., Jr., O'Leary, J.L., and Ferguson, J.P. (1966). The trigeminal, facial, vagal, and glossopharyngeal nerves in the monkey. *Arch. Neurol. 14*, 530–540.

Robertson, B., and Aldskogius, H. (1982). The use of anterogradely transported wheat germ agglutinin-horseradish peroxidase conjugate to visualize cutaneous sensory nerve endings. *Brain Res. 240*, 327–330.

Rustad, W.H., and Morrison, L.F. (1952). Revised anatomy of the recurrent laryngeal nerve. *Laryngoscope 62*, 237–249.

Sasaki, Y. (1943). Distribution of nerve fibers in the human larynx. *Tohoku Med. J. 32*, 569–594.

Sugano, M. (1929). Über die Kehlkopfnerven, experimentelle Untersuchungen über die Innervation des Kehlkopfes. *J. Otolaryngol. Jpn. 35*, 1138–1361.

Suzuki, M., and Kirchner, J. A. (1968). Afferent nerve fibers in the external branch of the superior laryngeal nerve in the cat. *Ann. Otol. Rhinol. Laryngol. 77*, 1059–1071.

Tomita, H. (1974). Fundamental matters of the taste. [Japanese]. *J. Otolaryngol. Jpn. 77*, 415–418.

Torvik, A. (1956). Afferent connections to the sensory trigeminal nuclei, the nucleus of the solitary tract and adjacent structures, an experimental study in the rat. *J. Comp. Neurol. 106*, 51–141.

Watanabe, S. (1985). Morphological investigation of sensory nerve endings of the human larynx. *Otologia (Fukuoka) 31*, 330–345.

Yatake, Y. (1965). Anatomical study on the laryngeal nerves of mammals. *Otologia (Fukuoka) 11*, 49–77.

Williams, A. F. (1954). The recurrent laryngeal nerve and the thyroid gland. *J. Laryngol. Rhinol. & Otol. 68*, 719–725.

CHAPTER 4

Sensory Nerve Endings of the Human Laryngeal Mucosa

Takemoto SHIN,
Shun WATANABE,
and Tadatsugu MAEYAMA

The three main functions of the larynx are phonation, respiration, and the protective reflex during deglutition. However, its primal function is sphincteric in nature. The sensory nerve endings in the laryngeal mucosa play an important role in reflex closure of the larynx. Several investigations on the structure of sensory nerve endings of the human laryngeal mucosa have been reported, but their role in the physiological function of the larynx has not been described as yet in detail. On the other hand, it appears that clinical features resulting from disturbance in the protective reflex are attributed to pathological changes of the peripheral sensory nerve. For example, aspiration due to recurrent laryngeal nerve paralysis in adults and frequent foreign body aspiration in infants under 2 years of age have been thought to result from disturbances in this reflex. This study was carried out to examine the structure of the sensory nerve endings of the human laryngeal mucosa, by means of light and electron microscopy. As mechanoreceptive sensory nerve endings seem to be most intimately related to the interaction between the nerve endings and surrounding tissues, ultrastructural investigation of these nerve endings is expected to contribute valuable information to the understanding of laryngeal function.

MATERIALS AND METHODS

Silver Impregnation

Specimens were surgically removed from four male patients

with laryngeal cancer, one female patient with hypopharyngeal cancer, and one male patient with tracheal cancer. None of the patients received radiation treatment prior to surgery. All specimens were taken from normal mucosa of the larynx, distant from the lesion. Also, four normal larynges were removed from a newborn infant, an 18 month old infant, a 6 year old child, and a 13 year old child at the time of autopsy. These specimens were used for silver staining only. The samples were fixed with ten percent formalin, washed in tap water, dehydrated with ethanol and embedded in paraffin. Sections 15 to 40 μm thick were cut and mounted on gelatin coated slides, which were placed in 40 ml of filtered 20 percent silver nitrate solution and put into an oven (60°C) for 15 min. They were then washed and placed in ammoniacal silver solution and ten drops of two percent formalin were added. Five to ten min were required for silver impregnation of the nerve fibers to be completed.

Electron Microscopy

Specimens were surgically removed from two patients suffering from laryngeal cancer. After excision, the lateral portion of each epiglottis was dissected out, cut into small pieces, and fixed in 2.5 percent glutaraldehyde in 0.1M phosphate buffer (pH 7.4) for two hr, and were then dehydrated with ethanol and embedded in epoxy resin. Sections of 1 μm thickness were cut and scanned for nervous elements in the subepithelial tissues after toluidine blue staining. Ultra thin sections were cut with a Porter-Blum ultramicrotome MT-1A and examined with a JOEL 1200 EX electron microscope after staining with both uranyl acetate and lead citrate.

RESULTS

Observation by Silver Impregnation

Findings in Adults

On the laryngeal surface of the epiglottis, nerve fascicles having myelinated or unmyelinated fibers were observed among the elastic and collagenous fibers. Fascicles of about 50 to 100 μm in diameter were observed about 300 to 600 μm below the epithelium. Peripheral nerve fibers separated from nerve fascicles extended upward vertically or obliquely toward the epithelium, finally making direct contact with basal cells of the epithelium and forming nerve endings (Figure 4-1). The type of nerve endings observed in this area were simple free endings (Figure 4-2), complex tree-like shaped endings (Figure 4-3), and corpuscular endings with glomerular pattern (Figure 4-4). Corpuscular endings were 5 to 150 μm in diameter. Several other fine terminal fibers, 0.1 to 0.2 μm in diameter, extended into the epithelial layer, branching from nerve endings.

In these structures, nerve varicosities of the terminal axon appeared not only under the epithelium but also in the epithelial layer. In the tree-like shaped endings, varicosities were observed at a turning point. The diameter of the varicosities was 3 to 6 μm under the epithelium and about 1 μm in the epithelial layer. In these varicosities, a glomerular pattern of fine neurofibrils was observed. In the laryngeal mucosa, sensory nerves and their endings were observed most frequently on the laryngeal surface of the epiglottis.

In the arytenoid region and the false fold, a comparatively large number of simple tree-like shaped endings and a small number of glomerular endings were observed under the basal cells of the epithelium. The glomerular endings were not strongly developed as in the epiglottis. Very small numbers of fine terminal fibers were observed in the epithelial layer.

In the vocal fold, a very few simple free endings were observed in the posterior region of the membranous portion and the density of elastic and collagenous fibers was much less than in the epiglottis.

Findings in a Neonate Infant

Nerve fascicles with myelinated or unmyelinated fibers on the laryngeal surface of the epiglottis were found somewhat less than in adults. However, a few nerve fascicles with myelinated or unmyelinated fibers were observed among areas rich in collagen and elastic fibers surrounding the epiglottic cartilage. Although several peripheral nerve fibers separated from nerve fascicles extended upward toward the epithelium, few were observed on the lingual surface of the epiglottis. On the laryngeal surface, a few

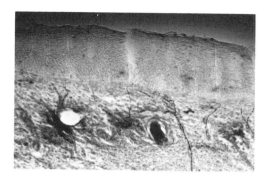

Figure 4-1. *A histological picture of free nerve endings in the laryngeal surface of the epiglottis of an adult male. Free nerve endings extend upward vertically or obliquely toward the epithelium. They make direct contact with basal cells of the epithelium.*

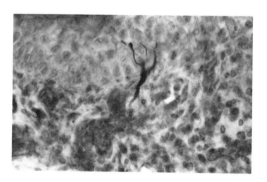

Figure 4-2. *A histological picture of simple free endings shown in the laryngeal surface of the epiglottis of an adult male. The type of nerve endings shown in this area are simple free endings.*

nerve fibers were observed reaching toward the epithelium. These were much less common than in adults, and complicated nerve networks and corpuscular nerve endings in the subepithelium nerve were observed (Figure 4-5). This same tendency was noted in the arytenoid and the false folds. The vocal folds were less developed in terms of nerve fibers and of fibrous tissue in the subepithelium.

Findings in Infants

The structure of the fasciculus and nerve endings in an 18 month old infant was found to have no remarkable variances from that of a neonate (Figure 4-6). However, the structure of nerve endings was fairly well developed in the 6 year old. In the 13 year old, it was quite similar to that of the adult (Figures 4-7, 4-8).

Observations by Electron Microscope

The present electron microscopic studies were confined to the laryngeal surface of the epiglottis because our light microscopic studies revealed that nerve fascicula and terminals were most densely distributed in this region.

In the nerve endings of the human epiglottis, the varicosity of the terminal axon made close contact with basal cells of the epithelium (Figure 4-9). The terminal axon was characterized by the presence of numerous mitochondria, many glycogen particles, synaptic-like vesicles, neurofilaments, and lysosomes (Figure 4-10). In the region where

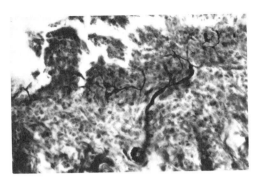

Figure 4-3. A histological picture of another type of nerve endings in the laryngeal surface of the epiglottis of an adult male. This type of nerve endings shows a complex tree-like shape.

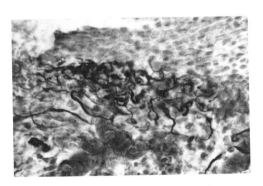

Figure 4-4. A histological picture of corpuscular nerve endings in the laryngeal surface of the epiglottis of an adult male. In this area, corpuscular endings with glomerular patterns can be seen.

the axons were in direct contact with the basal cells of the epithelium or the extracellular space, the Schwann cell sheath was often absent. The diameter of these varicosities varied from 3 to 6µm. No membrane specialization was observed between the nerve varicosities and the basal epithelium cells in the contact zone.

From some of the nerve varicosities protruded a process that was covered with a neuronal membrane, devoid of a Schwann cell sheath (Figure 4-11), and contained small clear vesicles, dense cored vesicles, and some glycogen particles. Thus, these nerve processes were not packed with mitochondria, but were packed with vesicular components instead.

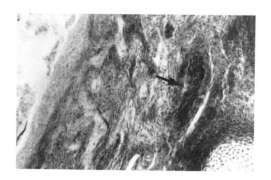

Figure 4-5. *A histological picture of the laryngeal surface of the epiglottis of a newborn infant. Complex nerve endings cannot be seen on the laryngeal surface of the epiglottis. Arrow indicates the nerve bundle adjacent to the cartilage.*

DISCUSSION

The reflex closure of the larynx is one of its most important functions, and sensory nerve endings of the laryngeal mucosa cause this reflex. Many neurophysiological investigations of the afferent discharges from the larynx (Andrew 1956; Sampson and Eyzaguirre 1964; Kirchner and Suzuki, 1968 Storey, 1968; Suzuki and Kirchner 1968, 1969; Morikawa, 1985) have been reported. However, the structure of these endings has not been elucidated in detail.

Silver impregnation is a very useful technique for observing the nerves and their endings. Sasaki and Matsumoto (1950) reported microscopic observation of the nerves and endings of the human laryngeal mucosa by means of

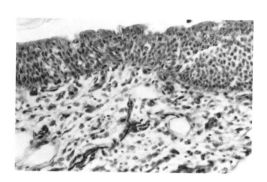

Figure 4-6. *A histological picture of the laryngeal surface of the epiglottis of an 18 month old child. The structure of the nerve ending indicates no remarkable variances from that of a newborn. At this age, numbers of myelinated fibers and nerve fibers extending toward the epithelium are slightly increased.*

Bierschowsky's method. Koenig and von Leden (1961a,b) reported an investigation of the peripheral nervous system of the human laryngeal mucosa with a modification of Bodian's method. We adopted a different technique, namely, Sevier and Munger's method (1965), for this investigation because it is more useful for observing details of the endings than Bierschowsky's method.

In our observations, peripheral terminal nerve fibers extended upward toward the epithelium from the nerve fascicula with myelinated and unmyelinated fibers. The types of sensory nerve endings observed in the laryngeal mucosa were free endings of simple and complex tree-like shape and corpuscular endings with a glomerular pattern. Several other fine terminal fibers extended into the epithelial layer. Highly developed endings similar to Pacini's corpuscle or Meissner's corpuscle were not observed. These structures were also reported by Sasaki (1943), Matsumoto (1950), and Koenig and von Leden (1961a,b) and our findings were inconsistent with their results. Koenig and von Leden assumed that the corpuscles were not receptors of specific sensations, but regulators of nerve stimuli. However, we regard the corpuscles as receptors because they make direct contact with basal cells of the epithelium.

In our investigation, nerves and their endings were observed most frequently on the laryngeal surface of the epiglottis. This finding is consistent with reports by Sasaki (1943). Hirano, Kurita, and Nakashima (1981) reported that in the superficial layer of the lamina

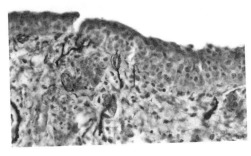

Figure 4-7. *A histological picture of the laryngeal surface of the epiglottis of a 6 year old child. The structure of the nerve endings is a developed complex tree-like shape similar to but not entered as far as those observed in adults.*

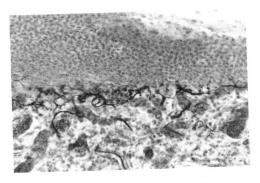

Figure 4-8. *A histological picture of the laryngeal surface of the epiglottis of a 13 year old child. On the laryngeal surface of the epiglottis numerous nerve endings can be seen quite similar in development to those of adults.*

propria of the vocal fold, elastic and collagen fibers are scarce. In this area, nerves and endings were very rarely seen. Nagai (1982) reported observing a corpuscle with a capsule (similar to Krause's corpuscle) in the subepithelial region of the vocal fold. However, we were unable to confirm the presence of corpuscles in this area.

The formation and development of the sensory nervous system of the larynx has been reported by Momono (1951) and Koenig and von Leden (1961a,b). They compared adults and fetuses from a morphological point of view. Development of the sensory nerve endings as they pertain to function was not discussed. Our results from infants indicate that the peripheral nerve fibers that branch from the nerve fasciculus increased upward toward the epithelium with age, finally making direct contact with basal cells of the epithelium by the age of 2 or 3 years. These data are consistent with the functional development of the laryngeal reflex. Therefore, we interpret these data to mean that development of the sensory nerves is one of the most important factors in development of the laryngeal protective reflex.

The present electron microscopic studies revealed the fine structure of the endings and the relationship between the endings and surrounding tissues. It is probable that we observed nerve varicosities of the glomerular corpuscle (Chiba, Watanabe, and Shin, 1985). These varicosities made close contact with basal cells of the epithelium and in the regions where they were in direct

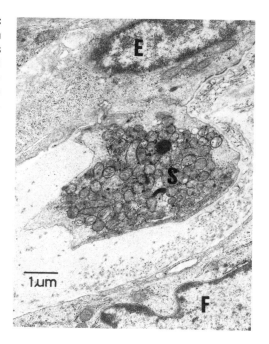

Figure 4-9. An electron micrograph demonstrating nerve endings in the laryngeal surface of the epiglottis of an adult male. The varicosity of the terminal axon (S) makes close contact with basal cells of the epithelium (E). Fibroblasts (F) are seen in the lower right corner.

contact with basal cells or extracellular space, the Schwann cell sheath was often absent. No membrane specializations were observed between the nerve varicosities and the basal epithelium cells in the contact zone. The structure of the endings is suitable for response to various degrees of stimulation, including weak stimulation. It is probable that the laryngeal mucosa, especially the laryngeal surface of the epiglottis, possesses fine sensitivity to stimulation.

SUMMARY

This study was carried out to examine the structure of sensory nerve endings of the human laryngeal mucosa by means of light and electron microscopy and to discuss their relationship to the physiological function of the larynx. The results are summarized as follows: (1) In adults, sensory nerves and their endings are observed most frequently on the laryngeal surface of the epiglottis. (2) A comparatively large number of sensory endings are seen in the arytenoid region and false fold, although they are not as strongly developed as in the epiglottis. (3) Sensory nerve endings are very rarely seen in the vocal folds. (4) The types of sensory nerve endings observed in this study are free endings of simple or complex tree-like shape and corpuscular endings with glomerular patterns. (5) In the terminal portion, some varicosities of the axon or concentration of the terminal fibers are observed under the epithelium.

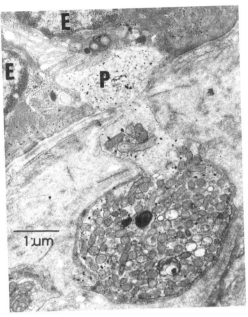

Figure 4-10. *An electron micrograph demonstrating nerve endings in the laryngeal surface of the epiglottis of an adult male. A process (P) devoid of a Schwann cell sheath in contact with the basal cells (E). Vesicles, glycogen particles, and tubular structure occupy the process.*

Moreover, very small varicosities of the fine terminal fibers are seen in the epithelium. (6) Using electron microscopy, nerve varicosities with an accumulation of mitochondria were observed. They partially lack the cytoplasm of Schwann cells and are in close contact with basal cells of the epithelium. No membrane specializations were observed between the basal epithelial cells and nerve varicosities.

ACKNOWLEDGMENTS

We are grateful to Professor Chiba, Department of Anatomy, Saga Medical School, for his guidance in electron microscopy. We would like to thank Mrs. Lisa Tsukamoto for her revision of the English.

This work was supported by Grant No. 59771212 from the Ministry of Education, Science, and Culture, Japan.

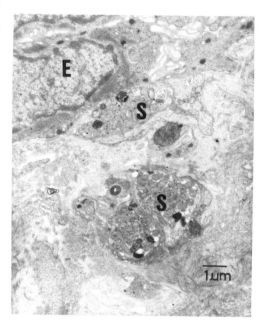

Figure 4-11. *An electron micrograph demonstrating nerve endings in the laryngeal surface of the epiglottis of an adult male. From some of the nerve varicosities (S) protrudes a process which is covered with a neuronal membrane and is devoid of a Schwann cell sheath. No membrane specializations can be seen between the nerve varicosities and basal epithelial cells (E).*

REFERENCES

Andrew, B.L. (1956). A functional analysis of the myelinated fibers of the superior laryngeal nerve of the rat. *J Physiol, 133*, 420–432.

Chiba, T., Watanabe, S., and Shin, T. (1985). Ultrastructure of the glomerular corpuscular nerve endings in the subepithelium of human epiglottis. *Arch Histol Jap, 45*, 145–153.

Hirano, M., Kurita, S., and Nakashima, T. (1981). The structure of the vocal folds. In K. N. Stevens and M. Hirano (Eds.), *Vocal fold physiology* pp. 33–41). Tokyo: University of Tokyo Press.

Kirchner, J.A., and Suzuki, M. (1968). Laryngeal reflexes and voice production. *Ann N Y Acad Sci, 155*, 98–109.

Koenig, W.F., and von Leden, H. (1961a). The peripheral nervous system of the human larynx. Part I. The mucous membrane. *Arch Otolaryngol, 73*, 21–34.

Koenig, W.F., and von Leden, H. (1961b). The peripheral nervous system of the human larynx. Part III. The development. *Arch Otolaryngol, 74*, 494-500.

Matsumoto, T. (1950). Innervation, especially sensory innervation of the laryngeal mucosa except the epiglottis. *Tohoku Igaku Zassi, 45*, 11–18.

Momono, T. (1951). Histological study of the nerve distribution of the larynx in human fetus. *Tohoku Med J, 46*, 102–109.

Morikawa, I. (1985). Basic investigation of the mechanism of the aspiration caused by recurrent laryngeal nerve paralysis during deglutition. *OTOLOGIA FUKUOKA, 31*, 315–329.

Nagai, T. (1982). Encapsulated sensory corpuscle in the mucosa of human vocal cord: An electron microscope study. *Arch Histol Jap, 45*, 145–153.

Sampson, S., and Eyzaguirre, C. (1964). Some functional characteristics of mechanoreceptors in the larynx of the cat. *J Neurol, 27*, 464–480.

Sasaki, Y. (1943). Microscope observation of the innervation of the human larynx. *Tohoku Igaku Zassi, 32*, 569–594.

Sevier, A.C., and Munger, B.L. (1965). A silver method applicable to paraffin sections of the formalin fixed tissue. *J Neuropath Exp Neurol, 24*, 130–135.

Storey, A. T. (1968). A functional analysis of sensory units innervating epiglottis and larynx. *Exp Neurol, 20*, 366–383.

Suzuki, M., and Kirchner, J. A. (1968). Afferent nerve fibers in the external branch of the superior laryngeal nerve in the cat. *Ann Otol, 77*, 1059–1070.

Suzuki, M., and Kirchner, J. A. (1969). Sensory fibers in the recurrent laryngeal nerve. *Ann Otol, 78*, 21–31.

CHAPTER 5

Autonomic Innervation of the Canine Larynx

Yasuo HISA
and Fumihiko SATO

Although the autonomic component would appear to be an important element in laryngeal innervation, investigations directed toward the laryngeal autonomic system have rarely been reported. The present study was undertaken with two objectives: (1) to clarify the noradrenergic (NA) innervation of the larynx by fluorescence histochemistry (Flack, Hillarp, Thieme, and Trop, 1962), and (2) to investigate the participation of the substance P (SP), one of the neuropeptides, in laryngeal autonomic innervation, using peroxidase-anti-peroxidase (PAP) immunohistochemistry.

MATERIALS AND METHODS

Dogs were used as experimental animals and were anesthetized by an intramuscular injection of ketamine (30 mg/kg).

At the end of the operation they were sacrificed. Two days before laryngectomy, each laryngeal nerve was crushed at the level where it enters the larynx to allow for accumulation of NA fluorescent material and SP immunoreactive material. In some dogs, the origin and course of NA fibers within each nerve were examined surgically before laryngeal extirpation.

Fluorescence Histochemistry

After laryngectomy, tissues were immediately frozen in isopentane-dry ice, and freeze-dried in vacuo at -40°C for five days. They were then exposed to paraformaldehyde for one hr at 80°C and embedded in paraffin. Sections (8 μm thick) were cut and mounted in Entellan-xylene mixture and examined by fluorescence microscopy.

PAP Immunohistochemistry

Each animal was perfused with 2 litres of ice-cold phosphate-buffered saline (PBS; 0.1M phosphate buffer, 0.9 percent NaCl, pH 7.4) followed by 3 litres of an ice-cold fixative containing 4 percent paraformaldehyde, 0.3 percent glutaraldehyde and 0.2 percent picric acid in 0.1M sodium phosphate buffer (PB; pH 7.4). After perfusion, the tissues were removed and postfixed for 48 hr at 4°C in a fixative containing 4 percent paraformaldehyde and 0.2 percent picric acid, buffered with PB. The fixed specimens were immersed in PB containing 15 percent sucrose for 48 hr at 4°C. They were sectioned at $2\mu m$ on a cryostat. These sections were processed for immuno-histochemistry according to the method reported by Kimura, McGeer, Peng, and McGeer (1981). The unlabeled antibody PAP developed by Sternberger (1979) was also used. Free-floating sections were pretreated with 0.3 percent Triton X-10 for four days and treated with 0.1 percent normal bovine serum for one hr, then incubated for five days with anti-SP serum (dilution x 5000, obtained from Immuno Nuclear Corporation). They were then incubated with anti-rabbit IgG (Miles; 1:200) for two hr, and with PAP complex (Dako; 1:200) for two hr at room temperature. Sections were washed in PBS containing 0.3 percent Triton X-100 before they were transferred from one serum to another. They were next incubated in a solution containing 0.02 percent 3,3′ diaminobenzidine and 0.015 percent H_2O_2 for ten min at room temperature.

Finally, they were mounted on chrome-coated glass slides, air dried, and washed with tap water. These sections were dehydrated in a graded series of ethanol, then cleaned in xylene with Entellan. As a control, some sections were treated with anti-SP serum absorbed with synthetic SP (50mɳ/ml). Positive immunoreactivity was not detected in the control sections.

RESULTS

NA nerve fibers were detected as greenish fluorescent fibers in the sections studied by fluorescence histochemistry and SP nerve fibers as brown immunoreactive fibers in the group studied by PAP immunohistochemistry.

Laryngeal Mucosa

NA nerve fibers were rarely observed in the epithelium and upper submucosa, although many isolated SP immunoreactive nerve fibers with varicosities were found. These SP fibers were situated between the epithelial cells (Figure 5-1A) and in the sub-epithelial connective tissue. Some of the SP fibers in the connective tissue were clearly associated with blood vessels (Figure 5-1B). Although SP is usually regarded as a primary sensory transmitter (Otsuka, Konishi, and Takahashi, 1975; Otsuka and Konishi, 1976), it is well known that SP exists in the autonomic nervous system (Wharton, Polak, McGeer, Bishop, and Bloom, 1981). SP nerve fibers located within the epithelium are free sensory nerve fibers and have no relationship to the autonomic innervation. But the existence of SP fibers associated with blood vessels suggests that SP also participates in the regulation of laryngeal blood flow volume.

Submucosal Glands

Many glands were observed in the submucosa of the epiglottis, ventricle, and subglottis. NA fibers were seen in the vicinity of the glands, but not within them. Some fibers with varicosities surrounded the base of these glands. Blood vessels in the connective tissue between the glands were also innervated by the NA fibers (Figure 5-2A).

Laryngeal secretion is essential to the lubrication of the vocal fold and to the immunological resistance of the larynx mucosa (Otsuka et al., 1975; Mogi, Watanabe, Maeda, and Umehara, 1979). Excitatory parasympathetic innervation of the laryngotracheal glands was identified by physiological techniques (Johnson, 1935) and the possibility of autonomic innervation of the laryngeal glands was suggested on the basis of morphology (Ardouin and Maillet, 1965; Armstrong and Hinton, 1951). On the other hand, sympathetic innervation of the laryngeal glands has not been detected. The present results strongly suggest the existence of NA innervation of the laryngeal glands.

A few isolated SP immunoreactive nerve fibers with varicosities were found in the subglottic regions. Some of these fibers appeared to terminate in glandular

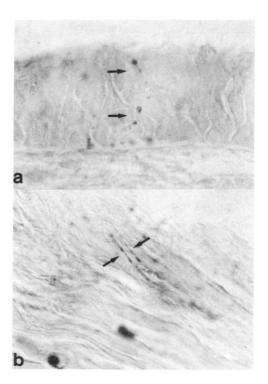

Figure 5-1. *A: SP immunoreactive nerve fiber with varicosities (→) observed within the subglottic epithelium (×810). B: SP immunoreactive nerve fibers with varicosities (→) associated with blood vessel in the connective tissue under the epithelium (×243).*

cells (Figure 5-2B), whereas others were observed to course parallel with blood vessels.

Uddman, Alumets, Densert, Hakanson, and Sundler (1978) reported that vasoactive intestinal polypeptide (VIP) participates in stimulating the secretory activity of the laryngeal glands. The present findings indicate the possibility that SP might be also involved in regulating laryngeal secretion. The report that SP nerve fibers were observed in relation to secretory elements in the salivary glands and the nasal mucosa also supports this idea (Hökfelt, Johansson, Kellerth, Ljungdahl, Nilsson, Nygards, and Pernow,1977).

Intrinsic Laryngeal Muscles

Many NA fibers were observed around the blood vessels in the intrinsic laryngeal muscles (Figure 5-3A). NA fibers that have no identifiable relationship to blood vessels were also observed running parallel with muscle fibers (Figure 5-3). SP nerve fibers were not observed in the intrinsic laryngeal muscles.

The dense population of NA fibers surrounding blood vessels in the intrinsic laryngeal muscles suggests the existence of a flow-regulating sympathetic innervation.

The existence of a direct sympathetic innervation of the intrinsic laryngeal muscles, blood vessels, and glands has been suggested by several investigators (Hartenau and Schwetz, 1956; Arnold, 1959). The present finding that many NA fibers run parallel with the muscle fibers, unrelated to blood vessels, supports this idea.

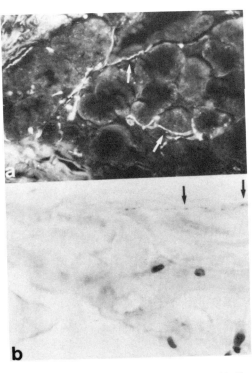

b

Figure 5-2. A: NA nerve fibers observed in the submucosal gland. Some fibers with varicosities surrounded the base of glands (→) (×260). B: SP immunoreactive nerve fiber with varicosities (→) observed to surround the submucosal gland (×243).

Laryngeal Nerves

NA Nerve Fibers

In cross sections, greenish fluorescent material was observed proximal to the crushing point in the external branch (SLNE) and the internal branch (SLNI) of the superior laryngeal nerve (SLN) and the recurrent laryngeal nerve (RLN).

Many investigators have reported that the laryngeal nerves contain many unmyelinated fibers (Heinbecker and O'Leary, 1933; Suzuki, 1935; Lemere 1932a; Lemere 1932b; Evans and Murray, 1954; Pressman and Kelemen, 1955; Gacek and Lyon, 1976). However, the existence of sympathetic nerve fibers in the laryngeal nerve has not been definitely clarified. Accumulation of catecholamine fluorescent material was demonstrated in the ligated or crushed peripheral nerves by fluorescence histochemistry and it was postulated that the fluorescent material revealed the preterminal axon of NA neurons (Dahlstrom and Fuxe, 1964; Dahlstrom, 1965). The catecholamine fluorescent material observed at the point proximal to the crushed portion of the laryngeal nerves shows NA fibers in each laryngeal nerve. All laryngeal nerves apparently act as channels for many postganglionic fibers of sympathetic nerves, along with the motor and sensory nerves.

The RLN was found to be composed of two similar-sized bundles. One bundle contained fluorescent material in abundance, whereas the other contained very little (Figure 5-4A). It is well known that the RLN usually divides into

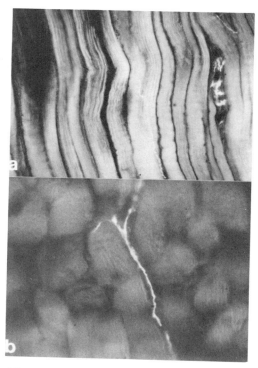

Figure 5-3. *A: Many NA nerve fibers were around the blood vessels and running parallel to the muscle fibers (×135). B: NA nerve fiber observed to run parallel to muscle fiber (×675).*

two main bundles before entering the larynx and that the posterior branch joins a branch of the SLNl, forming Galen's anastomosis (Dilworth, 1921; Lemere 1932a; Lemere 1932b; Armstrong and Hinton, 1951; Bowden, 1955; Harrison, 1981). In the experiments in which the anterior and posterior branches of the RLN were crushed, the posterior branch contained abundant fluorescent material. This fact confirms Lemere's observation (Lemere, 1932b) that unmyelinated postganglionic sympathetic fibers enter the larynx through the "pararecurrent nerve." This nerve originates from the vagus near the origin of the RLN and passes upward in the tracheoesophageal groove to interdigitate with fibers coming from above. These observations indicate that most NA fibers in the RLN traverse the larynx within the nerve's posterior branch.

When the superior cervical ganglion (SCG) had been resected seven days preoperatively, or the vagus nerve had been resected just above the level of the middle cervical ganglion (MCG), there was an obvious reduction in the amount of fluorescent material in the posterior branch of the ipsilateral RLN . When both the SCG and the MCG, or the RLN at its lowest level in the neck, had been resected seven days previously, the flourescent material in the posterior branch of the ipsilateral RLN disappeared completely. Fluorescent material was still present in another branch of the SLN seven days after resection of the ipsilateral SCG, but it had completely disappeared after unilateral resection of both the ipsilateral SCG and MCG, or the RLN at its

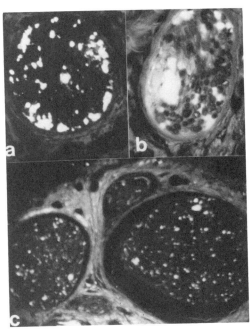

Figure 5-4. A: Cross section of the posterior branch of RLN (×135). B: Cross section of SLEN (×700). C: Cross section of SLNl (×110).

lowest level in the neck. Suzuki (Suzuki, 1935) consistently found one anastomotic branch between the MCG and the RLN in the dog. Nielsen, Owman, and Santini (1969) and Ohsumi, Tsunekawa, and Fujiwara (1974) reported that NA fibers originating from the SCG leave the sympathetic trunk and enter the vagus nerve below the level of the nodose ganglion (NG). These reports and the present study demonstrate that the RLN receives NA fibers not only from the SCG, but also from the MCG; and that NA nerve fibers originating from the SCG enter the RLN at its origin from the vagus nerve.

The SLNE carried one bundle which contained fluorescent material (Figure 5-4B). Seven days after SCG resection, this fluorescent material had completely disappeared from the ipsilateral SLNE. Cutting the SLN at its NG origin did not reduce the amount of fluorescent material in the ipsilateral SLNE. The SLNI was composed of three or four bundles of various sizes, all containing scattered fluorescent material (Figure 5-4C). Seven days after resection of the SCG, fluorescent material had completely disappeared from the ipsilateral SLNI. Fluorescent material in the SLNI showed no change after the ipsilateral SLN was cut at its NG origin.

Mitchell (1954) stated that post-ganglionic fibers from the SCG may join the SLN directly, but that they frequently pass through the pharyngeal plexus and therefore enter the larynx indirectly. The present study neither confirms nor disproves this observation. How-ever, it is certain that NA fibers enter the SLN after it leaves the vagus nerve, as fluorescent material is still observed after the SLN is cut at its NG origin. Mitchell (1954) also reported that the sympathetic nerve supply to the larynx was carried by the internal and external branches of the SLN, and by the laryngeal branches of the superior and inferior thyroid arteries. He did not report any participation by the RLN. The existence of perivascular sympathetic innervation along the superior and inferior thyroid arteries was also reported by Hartenau and Schwetz (1956). To determine whether the laryngeal nerves are the only source of sympathetic nerve supply to the larynx, we studied the distribution of the NA fibers after resection of all laryngeal nerves . Removal of the laryngeal nerves (SLNE, SLNI, and RLN) without severance of the laryngeal arteries caused complete disappearance of fluorescent nerve fibers in the muscles and glands. This result rules out the existence of a sympathetic perivascular innervation.

SP Nerve Fibers

Accumulation of SP immunoreactivity was not observed at the point at which each nerve had been crushed. However, some individual SP nerve fibers were found in the RLN and the SLNI above the point of crushing.

The SP fibers in the larynx could not have originated in neurons of the NG and entered the larynx through the vagus-RLN-SLN complex. The vagus nerve has been reported to contain many SP nerve fibers originating in the NG (Lundberg, et al., 1978). The present study demonstrates that the RLN and the SLN also contain SP nerve fibers.

ACKNOWLEDGMENT

Some parts of this text have been published as original papers (Hisa, 1982; Hisa, Sato, Fukui, Ibata, and Mizukoshi, 1982; Hisa, Sato, Fukui, Ibata, and Mizukoshi, 1985).

REFERENCES

Ardouin, P., and Maillet, M. (1965). Étude des fibres nerveuses amyeliniques de la corde vocale. *Acta Otolaryngol, 59*, 225–223.

Armstrong, W.G., and Hinton, J.W. (1951). Multiple divisions of the recurrent laryngeal nerve. *Archs Surg, 62*, 532–539.

Arnold, G. E. (1959). Vocal rehabilitation of paralytic dysphonia. *Arch Otolaryngol, 70*, 444–453.

Bowden, R.E.M. (1955). The surgical anatomy of the recurrent laryngeal nerve. *Br J Surg, 43*, 153–163.

Dahlstrom, A. (1965). Observations on the accumulation of noradrenaline in the proximal and distal parts of peripheral adrenergic nerves after compression. *J Anat, 99*, 677–689.

Dahlstrom, A., and Fuxe, K. (1964). A method for the demonstration of adrenergic nerve fibers in peripheral nerves. *Z Zellforsch mikrosk Anat, 62*, 602–607.

Dilworth, T.F.M. (1921). The nerves of the human larynx. *J Anat, 56*, 48–52.

Evans, D.H.L., and Murray, J.G. (1954). Histological and functional studies on the fibre composition of the vagus nerve of the rabbit. *J Anat, 88*, 320–337.

Flack, B., Hillarp, N.-A., Thieme, G., and Trop, A. (1962). Fluorescence of catecholamines and related compounds condensed with formaldehyde. *J Histochem Cytochem, 10*, 348–354.

Gacek, R.R., and Lyon, M.J. (1976). Fiber components of the recurrent laryngeal nerve in the cat. *Ann Otol Rhinol Laryngol, 85*, 460–471.

Harrison, D.F.N. (1981). Fibre size frequency in the recurrent laryngeal nerves of man and giraffe. *Acta Otolaryngol, 91*, 383–389.

Hartenau, W., and Schwetz, F. (1956). Beobachtungen nach experimenteller recurrensdurchtrennung bei der Katze. *Arch Ohr-Nas-KehlkHeilk, 169*, 242–245.

Heinbecker, P. and O'Leary, J. (1933). The mammalian vagus nerve. A functional and histological study. *Am J Physiol, 106*, 623–646.

Hisa, Y. (1982). Fluorescence histochemical studies on the noradrenergic innervation of the canine larynx. *Acta Anat, 113*, 15–25.

Hisa, Y., Matsui, T., Fukui, K., Ibata, Y., and Mizukoshi, O. (1982). Ultrastructure and fluorescence histochemical studies on the sympathetic innervation of the canine laryngeal glands. *Acta Otolaryngol, 193*, 119–122.

Hisa, Y., Sato, F., Fukui, K., Ibata, Y., and Mizukoshi, O. (1985). Substance P nerve fibers in the canine larynx by PAP immunohistochemistry. *Acta Otolaryngol, 100*, 128–133.

Hökfelt, T., Johansson, O., Kellerth, J.O., Ljungdahl, A., Nilsson, G., Nygards, A., and Pernow, B. (1977). Immunohistochemical distribution of substance P. In U.S. von Euler and B. Pernow (Eds.), *Substance P* (pp. 117–145). New York: Raven Press.

Johnson, J. (1935). Effect of superior laryngeal nerves on tracheal mucus. *Ann Surg,* *101,* 494–499.

Kimura, H., McGeer, P.L., Peng, J.H., and McGeer, E.G. (1981). The central cholinergic system studied by choline acetyltransferase immunohistochemistry in the cat. *J* *Comp Neurol, 200,* 151–201.

Lemere, F. (1932a). Innervation of the larynx. I. Innervation of Laryngeal muscle. *Am J* *Anat, 51,* 417–473.

Lemere, F. (1932b). Innervation of the larynx. II. Ramus anastomoticus and ganglion cells of the superior laryngeal nerve. *Anat Rec, 54,* 389–407.

Lundberg, J.M., Hökfelt, T., Nilsson, G., Terenius, L., Rehfeld, J., Elde, R., and Said, S. (1978). Peptide neurons in the vagus, splanchnic and sciatic nerves. *Acta Physiol* *Scand, 104,* 499–501.

Mitchell, G.A.G. (1954). The autonomic nerve supply of the throat, nose and ear. *J Lar* *Otol, 68,* 495–516.

Mogi, G., Watanabe, M., Maeda, S., and Umehara, T. (1979). Laryngeal secretions, an immunochemical and immunohistological study. *Acta Otolaryngol, 87,* 129–141.

Nielsen, K.C., Owman, C., and Santini, M. (1969). Anastomosing adrenergic nerves from the sympathetic trunk to the vagus at the cervical level in the cat. *Brain Res, 12,* 1–9.

Ohsumi, K., Tsunekawa, K., and Fujiwara, M. (1974). Fluorescence histochemical studies on adrenergic nerve fibers in the vagus nerve of rat. In M. Fujiwara and T. Tanaka (Eds.), *Amine fluorescence histochemistry* (pp. 93–104). Tokyo: Igaku Shoin.

Otsuka, M., Konishi, S., and Takahashi, T. (1975). Hypothalmic substance P as a candidate for transmitter of primary afferent neurons. *Fed Proc Fedn Am Soc Exp Biol, 34,* 1922–1928.

Otsuka, M., and Konishi, S. (1976). Release of substance P-like immunoreactivity from isolated spinal cord of newborn rat. *Nature, 264,* 83–84.

Pressman, J.J., and Kelemen, G. (1955). Physiology of the larynx. *Physiol Rev, 35,* 506–554.

Sternberger, L.A. (1979). *Immunocytochemistry* (2nd ed.). New York: J. Wiley.

Suzuki, S. (1935). Uber die Beziehungen zwischen dem Vagus und dem Sympathicus. *Tokyo Igaku Zassi, 49,* 1659–1675.

Uddman, R., Alumets, J., Densert, O., Hakanson, R., and Sundler, F. (1978). Occurrence and distribution of VIP nerves in the nasal mucosa and tracheobronchial wall. *Acta* *Otolaryngol, 86,* 443–448.

Wharton, J., Polak, J.M., McGeer, G.P., Bishop, A.E., and Bloom, S.R. (1981). The distribution of substance P-like immunoreactive nerves in the guinea-pig heart. *Neuroscience, 6,* 2193–2204.

Wyke, B.D., and Kirchner, J.A. (1976). Neurology of the larynx. In R. Hinchcliffe and D. Harrison (Eds.), *Scientific foundation of otolaryngology* (pp. 546–574). London: Heinemann.

CHAPTER 6

Substance P Immunoreactive Nerve Fibers of the Canine Laryngeal Mucosa

Takemoto SHIN,
Shigeru WADA,
and Tadatsugu MAEYAMA

Many investigations on substance P (SP) have recently been reported. At present, SP is considered a neurotransmitter. It is generally accepted that SP exists in sensory and autonomic nerve fibers. The purpose of this study is to correlate the immuno-histochemical features of SP with its distribution in the laryngeal mucosa. Using silver impregnation of the canine laryngeal mucosa, we studied the sensory nerve endings, laryngeal glands, and surrounding blood vessels by light and electron microscopy for SP immunoreactive nerve fibers (SP fibers).

MATERIALS AND METHODS

The larynx was surgically removed from ten mongrel dogs of both sexes weighing 8 to 10 kg and examined by three different techniques: silver impregnation, immunohistochemical, and electron microscopy.

Silver Impregnation

Specimens were resected from the canine laryngeal mucosa and fixed with neutral buffer formalin. Sections 30 μm thick were cut and stained with Gross-Schultze's method.

Immunohistochemical Technique of SP Fibers

After general anesthesia was induced with sodium pentobarbital (25 mg/kg), the bilateral carotid artery of each animal was perfused with 500 ml of heparinized physiological saline followed by two litres of an ice-cold fixative (Zamboni) containing 20 g of paraformaldehyde, 150 ml of saturated picric acid in one litre of 320 mOsM phosphate buffer (PB). After total laryngectomy, the specimens were postfixed for five hr at 4°C in the previously mentioned fixative. The fixed specimens were immersed in 0.01 M phosphate buffered saline (PBS) containing 20 percent sucrose for 48 hr at 4°C, then frozen in liquid nitrogen. Thirty μm sections were cut on a cryostat and mounted on PLL-coated slides. These were then pretreated with one percent hydrogen peroxide in methanol for five min, one percent normal saline serum for 30 min and incubated with anti-SP serum (1:1000 UCB Bioproducts) for less than 24 hr. They were then incubated with anti-rabbit IgG (1:50 Dako) for 45 min, and with PAP complex (1:80 Dako) for 45 min. The slides were thoroughly washed in 0.01M PBS before being transferred from one serum to the next. They were then incubated in a dark room in a buffer solution (20 mg 3.3′ diaminobenzidine in 100 ml Tris-buffer and 0.003 percent hydrogen peroxide) for nearly ten min at room temperature. The sections were then dehydrated in a graded series of ethanol, cleaned in xylene, and covered with Entellan. As a control, some sections were treated with normal rabbit serum (1:1000). Positive reactivity was not detected in the control sections.

Electron Microscopy

Zamboni's fixative was perfused through the bilateral carotid artery under general anesthesia with nembutal after ligation of the internal and external carotid arteries. The larynx was removed and immersed in the same fixative for six hr. The laryngeal membrane was then cut into blocks (approximately 2 × 4 × 5 mm) and washed several times in 0.01M PBS (pH 7.4). The sections were cut on a Vibratome, and immuno-cytochemical procedures were carried out in the same manner used for the light microscopy technique.

For the localization of peroxidase activity, sections were pre-incubated for not more than 15 min in 0.05 percent 3,3′-diaminobenzidine dissolved in 0.005 M Tris-HCl buffer, pH 7.4, containing 0.01 percent hydrogen peroxidase. The sections were then washed in Tris buffer, treated with 25 percent glutaraldehyde for one hr, washed in 0.1M PB, and then fixed in one percent OsO4 in PB for one hr. This was followed by dehydration in a series of alcohols and immersion in Spurr resin, then the samples were cured for two days at 70°C.

After examination by light microscopy, a small piece of the section was cut out and mounted on a block of Spurr resin. Ultrathin sections were cut and collected on 200 meshes. Electron-micrographs were taken with a JEOL 1200 EX electron microscope.

RESULTS

Observation by Silver Impregnation

In the canine laryngeal mucosa, free nerve endings of simple or complex tree-like shape, corpuscle endings with glomerular pattern, and intra-epithelial free endings and taste bud-like structures were observed. They were composed of thick and thin sensory nerve fibers varying in diameter from 3.0 to 6.0 μm (thick) and from 0.2 to 1.0 μm (thin). Sensory nerve endings were most frequently observed on the epiglottis. Large numbers of intraepithelial free endings were observed, whereas other endings were rarely seen. Unencapusulated corpuscles were observed in the mucosa of the epiglottis but were rarely seen in the vocal fold. Corpuscles were found to be associated with fibroblasts. Taste bud-like structures were observed mainly on the epiglottis, particularly on the laryngeal surface. There were only thin fibers found in contact with the taste bud-like structures.

Observations by Immuno-histochemical Technique

Sub- and Intra-Epithelium Regions

In this study, many SP immunoreactive nerve fibers with varicosities were observed in the mucosa of the epiglottis, particularly on the laryngeal surface. In addition, SP was contained only in thin fibers, never in thick fibers. In the epithelium, many SP fibers extended independently to the free surface of the epithelium (Figure 6-1), some branching out into one or two thin fibers. The development of these intra-epithelial free nerve endings was comparatively rich in the lower part of the epiglottis and adjacent to the aryepiglottic fold. There were also a few nerve endings that terminated in varicosities beneath the basal cell layer of the epithelium (Figure 6-2).

In addition to these free nerve endings, we found many taste bud-like structures in the epithelium. There were two types of the terminal state of intragemmal SP nerve fibers. One was a simple branched termination composed of one or two SP nerve fibers that ascended from the basement membrane (Figure 6-3A). The other was a plexus-like termination which showed a network of some SP nerve fibers in the taste bud-like structures (Figure 6-3B).

Under the basement membrane, we found nerve corpuscles that contained SP immunoreactive nerve fibers (Figure 6-4). These corpuscles were nonencapsulated and were constituted from thin, reticulated fibers and some fibroblasts. SP immunoreactive nerve fibers originated from these corpuscles and were connected with free nerve endings and taste bud-like structures in the epithelium. The diameter of SP fibers varied from 0.2 to 0.8 μm.

Submucosal Glands

A few SP fibers were found in the submucosal glands. Varicosities were associated with gland cells (Figure 6-5). SP fibers with varicosities were observed to enter the glands, parallel with blood vessels.

Blood Vessels

SP fibers with varicosities were observed to course parallel to the blood vessels. Fine SP fibers were found to enter into the smooth muscle layer making varices at this site (Figure 6-6). The diameter of the blood vessels accompanied by SP fibers was larger than 30 μm. SP fibers were not found in the capillaries.

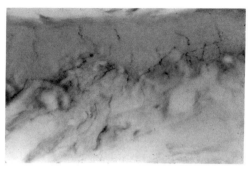

Figure 6-1. *Many SP fibers can be seen extending independently to the free surface in the epithelium of the canine laryngeal mucosa.*

Observations by Electron Microscopy

In the present study, the SP fiber of the vocal fold was observed by electron microscopy. The varicosity of the terminal axon made close contact with basal cells of the epithelium. No membranous specialization was observed between the nerve varicosities and the basal epithelial cells in the contact zones. Postsynaptic cells were not found. The fine structures were not clear because they were slightly damaged during immunoreaction. The reaction products seemed to be present in both the laryngeal vesicles and in the cytoplasm at the terminal axon. Some of the nerve varicosities extended a process which was covered with neuronal membrane, but devoid of a Schwann cell sheath (Figure 6-7). Terminal axons were found between the basal cells or in the hollow on the surface of the basal cells (Figure 6-8).

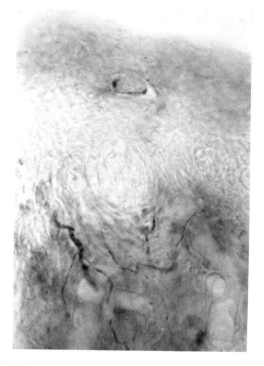

Figure 6-2. *Some SP fibers can be seen branching into one or two thin fibers in the intra-epithelial free nerve endings. There are also a few nerve endings that terminate in varicosities beneath the basal cell layer of the epithelium.*

DISCUSSION

Many investigations of sensory nerve endings of the laryngeal mucosa with silver impregnation have been reported (Sasaki, 1943; Matsumoto, 1950; Koizumi, 1953a,b; Koenig and von Leden, 1961; Watanabe, 1985), the results of which are consistent with our findings. Nagai (1982) reported an encapsulated corpuscle of the subepithelial region of the vocal fold. However, in our observations, an encapsulated corpuscle was not observed in the laryngeal mucosa. Highly developed endings similar to Pacini's corpuscle or Meissner's corpuscle were not observed. It has been established that SP is widely distributed in the peripheral nervous system (Hökfelt et al., 1977). It has also been shown by Ninoyu and colleagues (1983) (guinea pig) and Hisa and colleagues (1985) (dog) that SP is contained in thin nerve fibers (A, C). In our observation, SP fibers of the canine laryngeal mucosa were found under and in the epithelium, in the submucosal glands, and in the blood vessels.

Sensory Nerve Endings

Ninoyu et al (1983) and Hisa et al (1985) reported that SP was present in free nerve endings in and under the epithelium. In the present study we have demonstrated the presence not only of free endings but also of corpuscles and taste bud-like structures associated with SP. Silver impregnation studies revealed the existence of thick and thin fibers in sensory nerve endings. The

A

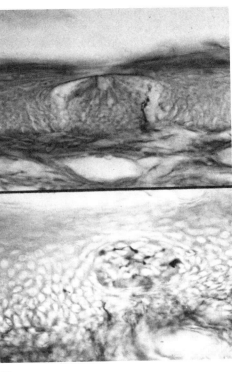

B

Figure 6-3. *Many taste bud-like structures can be seen in the epithelium. There were two types of the terminal state of intragemmal SP nerve fibers. A (upper figure) shows a simple branched termination composed of one or two SP nerve fibers which ascend from the basement membrane. B (lower figure) shows a plexus-like termination of SP nerve fibers in taste bud-like structures.*

diameter of SP fibers varied from 0.2 to 0.8 μm. From these results, it is suggested that SP was contained only in thin fibers. Hockfelt et al (1977) reported that SP was observed both in laryngeal granular vesicles and more diffusely in cytoplasm of central nerve endings. From our electron microscopic observations it is apparent that SP is contained in both large vesicles and cytoplasm at the terminal axon.

What physiological functions the SP fibers in the laryngeal mucosa may have are still unknown. Hökfelt et al (1977) reported that free nerve endings in the skin penetrating into the epithelium contained SP. Kennis et al (1984), reported that neurogenic plasma extravasation from the venules was evoked by polymodal nonreceptive C fibers and was likely, at least in part, to be mediated by SP. Possibly, one of the functions of the SP- containing free nerve endings of the laryngeal mucosa is to regulate the permeability of blood vessels through reflex pathways. However, SP fibers were not observed in venules of the laryngeal mucosa. Olgarth (1977) demonstrated that SP can be released from the peripheral sensory branch of tooth pulp and Hökfelt et al (1980), suggested that SP may function at its terminal branch by modulating the threshold of 'its own nerve'' endings. However, in the present study, electron microscopic observations failed to clarify whether or not SP was released from the terminal axon.

Physiologically, taste bud-like structures have been considered to function as receptors of taste

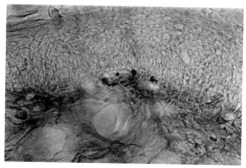

Figure 6-4. *Under the basement membrane, nerve corpuscles containing SP immunoreactive nerve fibers are shown.*

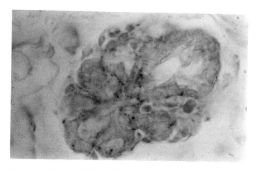

Figure 6-5. *A few SP fibers are shown in the submucosal glands. Varicosities are associated with gland cells.*

and/or receptors of pressure or touch (Koizumi, 1953a,b). Suzuki and Takeda (1983) observed taste buds in the epiglottis by electron microscopy and reported cholinergic fibers in contact with type I and type II cells of the taste bud. However, the neurotransmitter in the fiber which made synapse with type III cells was unknown. In the present study, we confirmed the presence of SP fibers in all taste bud-like structures of the epiglottis, but the types of taste bud-like structure were not identified. Hökfelt and colleagues (1980) reported that neuropeptide and classical neurotransmitters coexisted in many neurons. It may be that SP and acetylcholine coexist in nerve fibers of the taste bud-like structures. It is well known that the structural integrity of the taste bud is dependent on sensory nerves (Zalewski, 1973). Hockfelt and colleagues reported that SP may be of trophic importance for the structural integrity of the taste bud.

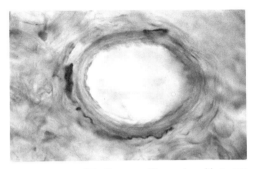

Figure 6-6. SP fibers with varicosities are shown extending parallel to blood vessels. Fine SP fibers were observed entering into the smooth muscle layer making varices at this site.

Submucosal Glands

SP fibers have commonly been observed in various glands. Hockfelt and colleagues (1980) reported that in the salivary glands and in the nasal mucosa SP fibers were associated with secretory elements. Ninoyu and colleagues (1983) and Hisa and colleagues (1985) reported that SP fibers were observed in the submucosal glands of the canine larynx. In our study, SP fibers were observed in association with gland cells. The lack of SP fibers in the submucosal glands suggests that they mainly innervate either serous or mucous glands.

Uddman and colleagues (1981) reported that vasoactive intestinal polypeptide (VIP) participates in stimulating secretory activity. Hökfelt and colleagues (1980) suggested that in the sweat glands, acetylcholine and VIP are released from the same nerve. Due to technical limitations, we were unable to determine whether SP and classical transmitters coexisted in the same nerve fiber. It is suggested that SP was released from the varicosities and that SP regulates laryngeal secretion in coordination with classical transmitters.

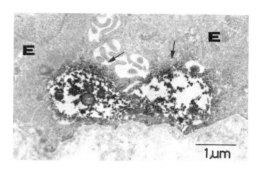

Figure 6-7. *Right arrow indicates that the terminal axon made close contact with basal cells of the epithelium (E). The reaction products appear to be present both in large vesicles and in the cytoplasm at the terminal axon. Arrow at left indicates that from some of the nerve varicosities extended a process which was covered with neuronal membrane, devoid of a Schwann cell sheath.*

Blood Vessels

It is also well known that SP fibers are found in association with blood vessels. Lembeck (1983) and Kennis and colleagues (1984) reported that injection of SP evoked cutaneous vasodilation and extravasation because the blood vessels are innervated with adrenergic and cholinergic fibers. We propose that SP acts as a regulator of contraction and permeability of the laryngeal mucosal arterioles in coordination with classical transmitters.

SUMMARY

This study was carried out to investigate the structure of sensory nerve endings and SP fibers of the canine laryngeal mucosa by means of light and electron microscopy. The results are summarized as follows:

1. Free nerve endings, corpuscular endings, and taste bud-like structures were observed.
2. Endings were composed of thin and thick nerve fibers.
3. SP was observed in nerve endings.
4. SP fibers were found to be related to the submucosal glands and blood vessels.
5. In the terminal axon of the sensory nerve, SP was found in large vesicles and cytoplasm.
6. SP fibers may be associated with reflex, secretory, and circulatory regulation in the larynx.

ACKNOWLEDGMENT

We would like to thank Mrs. Lisa Tsukamoto for her English revision in the preparation of this manuscript.

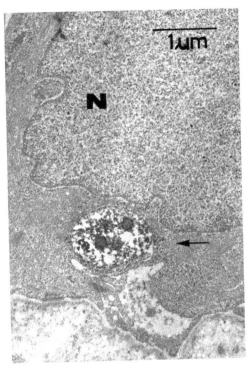

Figure 6-8. *Terminal axon (arrow) is shown between the basal cell or in the hollow on the surface of the basal cells. 'N'' indicates epithelial cell nucleus.*

REFERENCES

Hisa, Y. Sato, F., Fukui, K., Ibata, Y., and Misukoshi, O. (1985). Substance P nerve fibers in the canine larynx by PAP immunohistochemistry. *Acta Otolaryngol (Stockh), 10,* 128–133.

Hökfelt, T., Johansson, O., Kellerth, J.O., Ljungdahl, A., Nilsson, G., Nygards, A., and Pernow, B. (1977). Immunohistochemical distribution of substance P. In U.S. von Euler and B. Pernow (Eds.), *Substance P* (pp. 117–145). New York: Raven Press.

Hökfelt, T., Johansson, O., Ljungdahl, A., Lundberg, J.M., and Schultz, M. (1980). Peptidergic neurons. *Nature, 284,* 515–521.

Kennis, P., Hurley, J.V., and Bell, C. (1984). The role of substance P in the axon reflex in the rat. *Brit J Dermatol, 111,* 551–559.

Koizumi, H. (1953a). On sensory innervation of larynx in dog. *Tohoku J Exp Med, 58,* 199–210.

Koizumi, H. (1953b). On innervation of taste-bud in larynx in dog. *Tohoku J Exp Med, 58,* 211–215.

Koenig, W.F., and von Leden, H. (1961). The peripheral nervous system of the human larynx. Part 1, The mucosa membrane. *Arch Otolaryngol, 73,* 21–34.

Lembeck, F. (1983). Modification of vasodilation in the skin. *Brit J Dermatol, 109,* 1–9.

Matsumoto, T. (1950). Innervation especially sensory innervation of the laryngeal mucosa except the epiglottis. *Tohoku Igaku Zasshi, 45,* 11–18.

Nagai, T. (1982). Encapsulated sensory corpuscle in the mucosa of human vocal cord. *Arch Histol Jap 45,* 145–153.

Ninoyu, O., et al. (1983). Immunohistochemical studies of peptidergic innervation in the field of otolaryngology. *Pract Otol (Kyoto), 76,* 3229–3240.

Olgarth, L. (1977). Release of substance P-like immunoreactivity from the dental pulp. *Acta Physiol Scand, 101,* 510–512.

Sasaki, Y. (1943). Microscopy on the innervation of the human larynx. *Tohoku Igaku Zasshi (Japan), 32,* 569–594.

Suzuki, Y., and Takeda, M. (1983). Ultrastructure and monoamine precusor uptake of taste buds in the pharynx, nasopalatine ducts, epiglottis and larynx of the mouse. *Acta Anat Nippon, 58,* 593–605.

Uddman, R., et al. (1981). Peptide containing nerves in the nasal mucosa. *Rhinology, 19,* 75–79.

Watanabe, S. (1985). Morphological investigation of sensory nerve endings of the human larynx. *Otologia Fukuoka, 31,* 330–345.

Zalewski, A.A. (1973). Regeneration of taste bud in tongue grafts after reinnervation by neurons in transplanted lumbar sensory ganglia. *Exp Neurol, 40,* 161–169.

CHAPTER 7

A Study of the Neuromuscular Junction of the Posterior Cricoarytenoid Muscle: Electron Microscopy, Histochemical Staining of Acetylcholinesterase, Autoradiography, and Fluorescent Staining of Acetylcholine Receptors

Takashi KANDA,
Toshio YOSHIHARA
Mitsutada MIYAZAKI,
Hiroshi NAGATA,
Minoru NOMOTO,
Toshio KANEKO
and Yuji YAKU

The posterior cricoarytenoid (PCA) muscle, the only muscle opening the glottis, plays an important role in phonetic and inspiratory functions. The PCA muscle is known to be innervated by the recurrent laryngeal nerve, and clinically we often encounter laryngeal nerve paralysis of various causes. Although there have been several studies concerning the intrinsic laryngeal muscles (Matzel and Vosteen, 1963; Kawano, 1968; Shagel and Hast, 1974; Malmgren and Gacek, 1981) and the motor end plates of these muscles (Rossi and Cortestina, 1964; Abo, 1975; Morales, Rama, and

Gayoso, 1980; Rosen, Malmgren, and Gacek 1983; Michael, Malmgren, and Gacek, 1985; Gambino, Malmgren, and Gacek, 1985), few ultrastructural and experimental studies on the motor end plate have been reported.

This is a preliminary study of the neuromuscular junction (NMJ) of the normal PCA muscle, and has been presented, in part, in our previous reports (Kanda, Yoshihara, Miyazaki, and Kaneko, 1983; Yoshihara, Kanda, Yaku, and Kaneko, 1984). We studied the localization of acetylcholine receptors (AChR) by fluorescent staining of snake neurotoxins (δ-bungarotozin [δ-BTX] and erabutoxin b [Eb]) and autoradiography of ^{125}I-labeled δ-BTX. Furthermore, we examined the NMJ of the normal PCA muscle by using histochemical techniques and electron microscopy to identify acetylcholinesterase (AChE).

MATERIALS

For a study of the normal NMJ of the PCA muscle, larynges of cats and of human subjects were used. Larynges were obtained from adult cats by surgical removal under Nembutal anesthesia. Human adult larynges were obtained by surgical removal from patients with lower pharyngeal or laryngeal cancer. Human fetal larynges of 17 and 23 weeks were obtained by miscarriage or stillbirth. After dissection of the intrinsic laryngeal muscles, the PCA muscles were removed and examined.

METHODS

Electron Microscopy

The muscles were fixed in a mixture of 4 percent paraformaldehyde and 2 percent glutaraldehyde in a cacodylate-buffered solution. After the muscle bundles had been teased out, they were incubated by the Cooper ferrocyanide method according to Karnovsky (1964) in order to visualize the localization of the motor end plates. After a brief incubation, the tissues were postfixed with 1 percent OsO_4, dehydrated in graded series of ethanol, and embedded in Epon 812. Thin sections were stained with uranyl acetate and lead citrate for short intervals and examined with a HU-12 electron microscope.

Histochemical Staining of AChE

The muscles were fixed with 2 percent glutaraldehyde in a cacodylate-buffered solution with 2 mM calcium acetate. AChE was visualized by incubation of the muscle in an acetylcholine solution according to Lewis and Shute (1964). Incubation was performed at 4°C for 50–60 min. Some samples were used for light microscopic observation. Others were postfixed in 1 percent OsO_4 and embedded in Epon 812 for electron microscopic study. Thin sections were stained with uranyl acetate and lead citrate.

Fluorescent Staining of AChR

Rhodamine-labeled Eb (TMR-Eb) was prepared according to

the method of Ishikawa and Shimada (1980). The conjugation of FITC and TMR to δ-BTX was carried out by following the procedure of Nakane and Kawaoi (1974). The specimens were observed under a fluorescence microscope.

Autoradiography of AChR

The muscles were fixed in 2.5 percent paraformaldehyde in 0.1M phosphate buffer, and rinsed through PBS. The tissues were saturated by incubating in ^{125}I-labeled δ-BTX for 2 hr. The tissues were rinsed again in PBS and refixed in glutaraldehyde buffered with 0.1M cacodylate. After the muscles were teased out, they were attached to a glass slide, coated with Sakura-NRM$_2$ emulsion, and exposed at 4°C for 7 days.

RESULTS

Electron Microscopic Findings in the Normal PCA Muscle

In the PCA muscle of the 17 week fetus, the axon terminal of the motor end plate contained quite a few spherical synaptic vesicles 50 nm in diameter, a few dense core vesicles, and mitochondria. The primary synaptic cleft was found, measuring approximately 100 nm between the axolemmal surface membrane and muscle surface membrane, and containing some granular substances of low electron density. The secondary synaptic cleft was not developed. The post-synaptic membranes were thickened or exhibited high electron density, in contrast to the axon membrane. Some coated vesicles were found attached to the post-synaptic membrane in the sarcoplasmic side (Figure 7-1).

In the 23 week fetus, synaptic vesicles of the axon terminal had increased in number. The secondary synaptic cleft was not yet developed (Figure 7-2).

In the adult PCA muscle, the axon terminal contained numerous synaptic vesicles 50-70 nm in diameter. Primary and secondary synaptic clefts were well developed and the distance between the pre- and post-synaptic membranes was 100 nm (Figures 7-3, 7-4).

In the cat PCA muscle, the NMJ was basically the same as that of the human adult except that the secondary synaptic cleft was less developed in the cat. The primary synaptic cleft measured approximately 50 nm between the axon membrane and muscle surface membrane. Synaptic vesicles were approximately 30 nm in diameter (Figure 7-5).

Histochemical Findings of AChE in the Normal PCA Muscles

By light microscopy, the singly innervated motor end plate (single-motor end plate) was demonstrated as a small dot located on each individual muscle fiber of the human adult, fetus, and cat. Multiply innervated motor end plates (multi-motor end plates) were not found in any of the PCA muscles. The end plates did not form a definite band but were scattered on the muscle fibers. The activity zones of 17 and 23 week fetal PCA muscles were small and rounded, and were approximately 30 μm in size (Figure 7-6). By comparison, they were not small and round, but elongated and infolded at the edges (Figures 7-7, 7-8, 7-9) in the cat and adult human PCA muscles.

Electron microscopically, the subneural apparatus of the fetal NMJ was filled with electron-dense products, which is evidence of AChE activity (Figure 7-2). In the PCA muscle of the human adult and cat, AChE activity was seen in primary and secondary synaptic clefts (Figures 7-3, 7-4, 7-10).

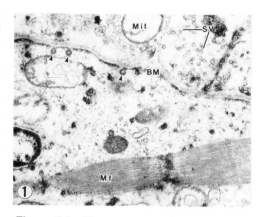

Figure 7-1. *The neuromuscular junction in the 17 week human fetal PCA muscle. The axon terminal contains numerous synaptic vesicles (SV), and a few coated vesicles (arrows) are attached to the postsynaptic membrane. Mitochondria (Mit), basement membrane (BM), myofibril (Mf). ×8650*

Localization of AChR in the Normal PCA Muscle

Fluorescent Staining of AChR by Using Eb and δ-BTX

These stainings were found at the NMJ where it is probably associated with the subsynaptic membranes. The neuromuscular localization of fluorescent staining was revealed by comparing phase contrast light microscopical findings (Figures 7-11, 7-12, 7-13).

[125]I-Labeled δ-BTX Binding

Autoradiography of ^{125}I-labeled δ-BTX showed that the grains lie especially at the junction folds. Radioactivity was distributed over a broad band coinciding with the junctional fold region (Figure 7-14).

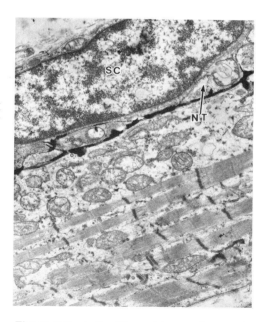

Figure 7-2. *In the 23 week human fetus, subneural apparatus is filled with electron-dense products, indicating AChE activity. Schwann cell (SC), nerve terminal (NT). ×6775.*

DISCUSSION

In this report we examined the NMJ of the PCA muscle by using various methods: electron microscopy, histochemistry of AChE, fluorescent staining of δ-BTX and Eb, and autoradiography of ^{125}I-labeled δ-BTX.

It is known that motor end plates of mammalian skeletal muscle are classified into two types according to the arrangement on the muscle fiber: (1) single-motor end plates, and (2) multi-motor end plates. They are also classified into three types by their structural differences: (1) en ligne type, (2) en grappe type, and (3) en plaque type. Rossi and Cortestina (1964) reported that multi-motor end plate fibers were found in 5 percent of the PCA muscles that they examined. In contrast, there are reports (Sonneson, 1960; Koenig and von Leden, 1961) that indicate that such fibers do not exist in the human laryngeal muscle. In the present study, only single-motor end plate and en plaque type NMJ were found in the human PCA muscle. Also, the end plates in the human PCA muscle did not form a definite band but were scattered on the muscle fibers. This scattered pattern is worth noting when considering the function of the PCA muscle.

In the PCA muscle of the 17 and 23 week fetuses, we observed AChE activity and an immature form of NMJ that was devoid of post-synaptic infoldings. Furthermore, the fact that we found some coated vesicles at the post-synaptic membrane was of interest. These coated vesicles may be involved in

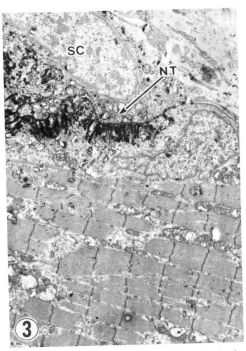

Figure 7-3. *The neuromuscular junction in the human adult. Intense reaction products are localized in the subneural apparatus. Schwann cell (SC), nerve terminal (NT).* ×5975

the transport of AChRs and of some other molecules.

For the histochemical staining of AChE, both Karnovsky's and Levis' methods were used. Electron microscopy using the former method showed coarse and non-homogeneous reaction products at the subneural apparatus of the MNJ, leading us to conclude that Levis' method is more appropriate for electron microscopy of the NMJ.

To identify the localization of AChRs, two kinds of snake toxin were used: δ-BTX and Eb, which are known to combine specifically with AChRs. In subsequent investigations we plan to study AChRs of the NMJ by using HRP-labeled Eb at the electron microscopic level.

ACKNOWLEDGMENT

We are very grateful to Professor Y. Shimada, Department of Anatomy, Chiba University, for helpful advice and encouragement during this presentation. The valuable assistance of Dr. Y. Ishikawa, Department of Anatomy, Chiba University, in producing this study, is gratefully acknowledged. We are indebted to Mr. N. Nakamura and Mrs. Shimizu for their technical assistance.

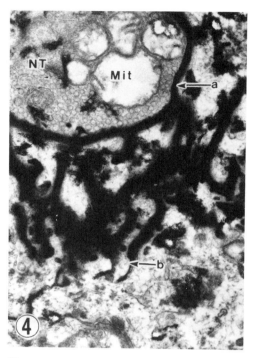

Figure 7-4. *High magnification of the neuromuscular junction in the human adult PCA muscle. AChE reaction products are seen in primary (a) and well developed secondary (b) synaptic clefts. × 13280*

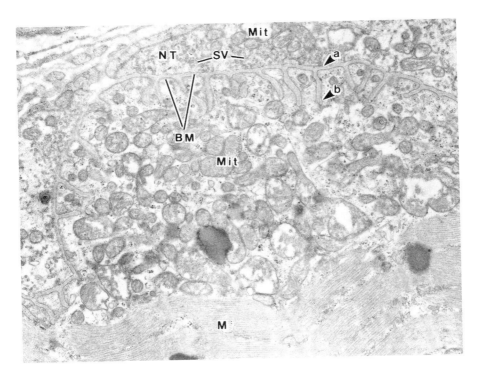

Figure 7-5. *An electron micrograph of the neuromuscular junction of the posterior cricoarytenoid muscle in the adult cat. Numerous synaptic vesicles (SV) and some mitochondria (Mit) are found in the terminal axon (NT). Primary synaptic cleft (a), secondary synaptic cleft (b), basement membrane (BM), myofibril (Mf). × 1560.*

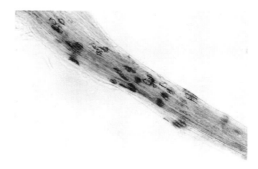

Figure 7-6. *A light micrograph of AChE activity in the 23 week human fetal PCA muscle according to the Lewis and Shute method. ×225.*

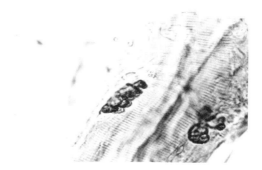

Figure 7-7. *AChE activity in the human adult PCA muscle. ×11250.*

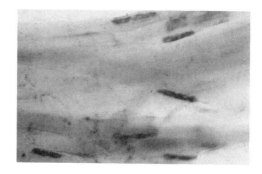

Figure 7-8. *A light micrograph of AChE activity in the adult cat PCA muscle according to Karnovsky's method. ×265.*

神経喉頭科学

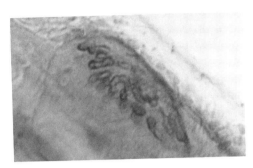

Figure 7-9. *High magnification of motor end plate. The subneural apparatus is clearly activated by AChE.* ×1800.

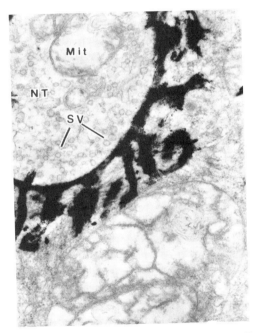

Figure 7-10. *Electron micrograph of AChE reaction in the adult cat PCA muscle. Note the subneural apparatus filled with electron-dense particles. Nerve terminal (NT), mitochondria (Mit), synaptic vesicle (SV).* ×12000.

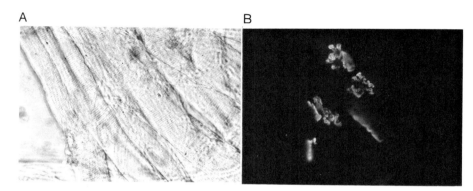

Figure 7-11. A: Phase contrast micrograph of the teased muscle fibers. ×500. B: Fluorescent staining with TMR-Eb. Note the array of the motor end plate on the same field of Figure 7-11a. ×415.

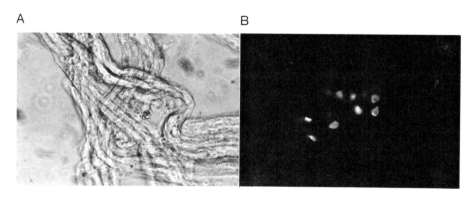

Figure 7-12. A: Phase contrast micrograph of the teased muscle fibers. ×340. B: Fluorescent staining with FITC-Eb on the same field of Figure 7-12A. ×282.

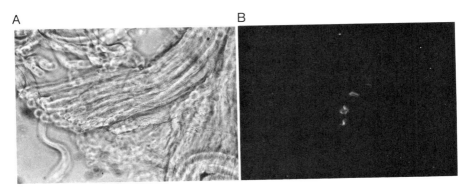

Figure 7-13. A: Phase contrast micrograph of the teased muscle fibers. ×282. B: Fluorescent staining with FITC-BT on the same field of Figure 7-13A. ×282.

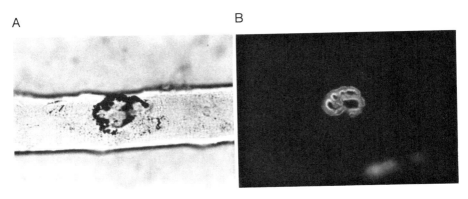

Figure 7-14. A: Localization on AChR by ¹²⁵I-labeled δ-BT binding at motor end palate. Note the accumulation of grains at the junctional folds. ×915. B: High magnification of fluorescent staining with FITC-BT. Note the remarkable activity at the junctional folds. ×915.

REFERENCES

Abo, El-Enene. (1975). Significance of the pattern of motor innervation of the intrinsic laryngeal muscles of cat. *Acta Anat, 93*, 543–553.

Gambino, D.R., Malmgren, L.T., and Gacek, R.R. (1985). Three-dimensional computer reconstruction of the neuromuscular junction distribution in the human posterior cricoarytenoid muscle. *Laryngoscope, 95*, 556–560.

Ishikawa, Y., and Shimada, Y. (1980). Fluorescent staining of acetylcholine receptors at the neuromuscular junction by means of rhodamine labeled erabutoxin b. In M. Ito, N. Tsukahara, K. Kubota, and K. Yagi (Eds.). *Integrative Congrol Functions of the Brain, Vol.III* (pp. 29–31). Tokyo: Elsevier/Kodansha Scientific.

Kanda, T., Yoshihara, T., Miyazaki, M. and Kaneko, T. (1983). Neuromuscular junctions of the posterior cricoarytenoid muscle in the cat. Fluorescent staining and autoradiography of acetylcholine receptors and histochemical staining of cholinesterase. *Acta Otolaryngol (Stockh), suppl 393*, 25–32.

Karnovsky, M.J., and Roots, L. (1964). A ''direct-coloring'' thiocholine method for cholinesterase. *J Histochem Cytochem, 12*, 219–221.

Kawano, A. (1968). Biochemical and electron microscopic investigation of the laryngeal muscles. *Otologia (Fukuoka) 14*, 306–343.

Koenig, W.F. and von Leden, H. (1961). The peripheral nervous system of the human larynx. II. The vocalis muscle. *Arch Otolaryngol, 74*, 153–163.

Lewis, P.R., and Shute, C.D. (1964). Demonstration of cholinesterase activity with electron microscope. *J Physiol (Lond), 175*, 5.

Malmgren, L.T., and Gacek, R. R. (1981). Histochemical characteristics of muscle fiber types in the posterior cricoarytenoid muscle. *Ann Otol, 90*, 423–429.

Matzel, D., and Vosteen, K.H. (1963). Electronoptische und enzymatische Untersuchungen des menschlicher Kehlkopf-muskulatur. *Arch Ohren Nasen Kehlkopf Heilkd, 181*, 447–457.

Michael, A.D.V., Malmgren, L.T., and Gacek, R.R. (1985). Three-dimensional distribution of neuromuscular junctions in human cricothyroid. *Arch Otolaryngol, 111*, 110–113.

Morales, J.R., Rama, J., and Gayoso, M. (1980). Some aspects of the nerve endings and synapses in the vocalis muscle. *J Laryngol Otol, 94*, 1047–1063.

Nakane, P.K., and Kawaoi, A. (1974). Peroxidase-labeled antibody. A new method of conjugation. *J Histochem Cytochem, 22*, 1084–1091.

Olgarth, L., Gazellus, B., Brodin, E., and Nilsson, G. (1977). Release of substance P-like immunoreactivity from the dental pulp. *Acta Physiol Scand, 101*, 510–512.

Rossi, G., and Cortestina, G. (1964). Morphological study of the laryngeal muscle of man. *Acta Otolaryngol (Stockh), 59*, 575–592.

Rosen, M., Malmgren, L.T., and Gacek, R.R. (1983). Three-dimensional computer reconstruction of the distribution of neuromuscular junctions in the thyroarytenoid muscle. *Ann Otol Rhinol Laryngol, 92*, 424–429.

Shagal, V., and Hast, M.H. (1974). Histochemistry of primate laryngeal muscles. *Acta Otolaryngol (Stockh), 78*, 277–281.

Sonesson, B. (1960). On the anatomy and vibratory pattern of the human vocal folds. *Acta Otolaryngol (Stockh), Suppl 156*, 1–80.

Yoshihara, T., Kanda, T., Yaku, Y., and Kaneko, T. (1984). Neuromuscular junctions of the posterior cricoarytenoid muscle in the human adult, human fetus and cat. Histochemical and electron microscopic study. *Acta Otolaryngol (Stockh), 97*, 161–168.

PART 2

Laryngeal Muscle

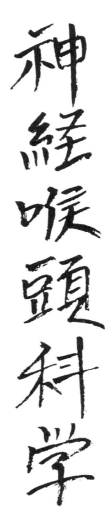

CHAPTER 8

A Histochemical Study of the Composition of Myosin and the Metabolic Enzyme Activities in Human Thyroarytenoid Muscle

Yasuo KOIKE
and Shinsaku NUNOMURA

The human thyroarytenoid muscle (TA) is highly specialized for phonation, but little is known about the histochemical basis of the physiological characteristics of various types of motor units in this muscle (Rosenfield, Miller, Sessions, and Patten, 1982). TAs contain a number of multiply innervated fibers (Bendiksen, Dahl, and Tei, 1981), but nothing is known about the physiological properties of these fibers. Multiply innervated skeletal muscle fibers that respond to stimulation by prolonged contraction rather than a twitch, so-called "slow tonic" fibers, are present in various classes of vertebrates (Hess, 1970), including human extraocular muscles (Dietert, 1965), where

they have been implicated in fixation and slow eye movements (Pierobon, Torresan, Sartore, Moschini, and Schiaffino, 1979).

Human TAs also differ from limb skeletal muscles in their structure (Rosenfield et al., 1982), neuromuscular junctions (Morales, Rama, and Gayoso, 1980), and histochemical reactions (Rosenfield et al., 1982). These morphological characteristics may be reflected in differences between the two types of muscles in patterns of morbidity and reactions in various neuromuscular disorders (Walton and Bardner-Nedwin, 1974).

No information is available on the myosin composition of multiply innervated fibers, and little is known about metabolic enzyme activities in muscle fiber types in the TAs. In the present study, we examined the histochemical characteristics of human TA fibers, in comparison with those of skeletal muscles.

MATERIALS AND METHODS

Muscle samples: Four specimens of TA, three specimens of extraocular muscle, and samples of various limb muscles were obtained at autopsy (2 to 4 hr after death) from four patients without any laryngeal or neuromuscular disorders. The specimens were immediately frozen in isopentane chilled with liquid nitrogen.

Immunohistochemical methods: Antimyosin antiserum raised against chicken slow tonic anterior latissimus dorsi (ALD) muscle and guinea pig slow twitch soleus (SOL) muscle myosin were kindly provided by Dr. Fujii (First Department of Pathology, Tokushima University). Immunostaining of serial transverse sections cut in a cryostat was carried out by the avidin-biotin-peroxidase compled (ABC) method (Hsu, Rainel, and Fanger, 1981).

Enzyme histochemistry: Serial sections alternating with those used for immunostaining were processed for examination of histochemical reactions. Sections were stained by histochemical methods for mysosin ATPase (pre-incubated at pHs 10.7, 4.65, 4.6, 4.4, 4.35) (Garnett, O'Donovan, Stephens, and Taylor, 1978), NADH-tetrazolium reductase (NADH-TR) (Dubuwitz and Brooke, 1973), menadione-linked alpha-glycerophosphate dehydrogenase (MAG) (Dubowitz and Brooke, 1973), phosphorylase (Meijer, 1968), and periodic acid-Schiff (PAS).

Neuromuscular junctions: Transverse serial sections of 10 μm thickness and longitudinal sections of 25 μm thickness were stained for acetylcholinesterase (AchE) (Koelle and Friedenwald, 1966), and counter-stained with Light Green.

RESULTS

The difference in myosin ATPase activities in TA fibers was similar to that between Type I and Type II fibers in skeletal muscles (Figure 8-1). The difference was most conspicuous when assayed at pH 10.7 and pH 4.35 (Figure 8-1): In fibers where ATPase activity was low at pH 10.7, the activity was generally high at pH 4.35 (Figure 8-1). Fibers with high ATPase activity at both pHs 10.7 and 4.35 were rare. In human limb muscles, Type IIA and Type IIB fibers can be clearly distinguished by their ATPase activity at pH 4.6 (Figure 8-3), but this was not so in the TA (Figure 8-1). NADH-TR activity was very high in TA fibers with acid-stable ATPase activity, and relatively high in TA fibers that resembled Type II limb skeletal muscle fibers in their ATPase activity (Figure 8-1). The MAG and phosphorylase activities and PAS reaction in TA fibers varied, and closely resembled those of human limb muscles (Figures 8-1, 8-2).

In various human skeletal muscles, anti-SOL stained all Type I fibers (Figure 8-1), that is, fibers

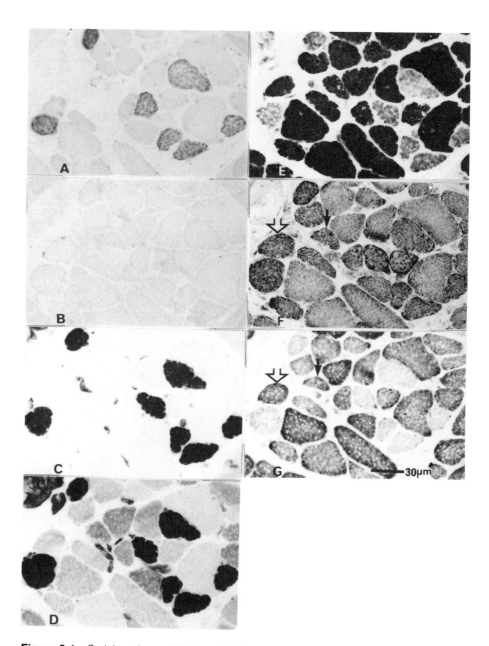

Figure 8-1. *Serial sections of TA. A: anti-SOL. B: anti-ALD. C: ATPase at pH 4.35. D: AT-Pase at pH 4.6. E: ATPase at pH 10.7. F: NADH-TR. G: MAG. Type II fibers (arrow-heads) show high NADH-TR and MAG activities.*

showing alkali-labile, acid-stable myosin ATPase activity (Figures 8-1,8-3). In contrast, anti-ALD stained only a few fibers in the extraocular muscles (Figure 8-4) and intrafusal muscles. Although multiply innervated fibers (both Type I and II) were present in the TA (Figures 8-5, 8-6, 8-7), like singly innervated limb muscle fibers, these fibers were not stained by anti-ALD. Fibers reacting with anti-ALD were mainly located in peripheral orbital layers (Figure 8-4). These fibers were also stained by anti-SOL, although often less intensely.

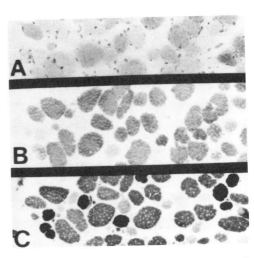

Figure 8-2. *Serial sections of TA. A: PAS. B: phosphorylase. C: ATPase at pH 4.65.*

DISCUSSION

This investigation showed the presence of two distinct types of slow fibers in human skeletal muscle differing in reactivity with anti-chicken ALD and anti-guinea SOL myosin. In contrast, in the TA, none of the fibers reacted with anti-ALD, but fibers with acid-stable myosin ATPase activity, whether with single or multiple innervation, reacted with anti-SOL. In the extraocular muscle, the fibers stained by anti-ALD showed acid-stable myosin ATPase activity.

Physiologic typing of slow fibers had led to the proposition of the existence of separate slow twitch and slow tonic contractile systems (Matyrushkin, 1961; Hess and Pilar, 1963; Mortensson and Skoglund, 1964; Bach-y-Rita and Ito, 1966). ALD muscle of chickens is composed of multiply innervated fibers that show slow tonic contraction (Ginsborg, 1960). Slow tonic fibers contract on treatment with succinylcholine, a property

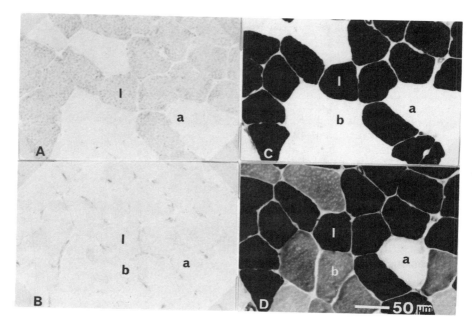

Figure 8-3. *Serial sections of gastrocnemius muscle. A: anti-SOL. B: anti-ALD. C: AT-Pase at pH 4.35. D: ATPase at pH 4.6. Fibers with intermediate ATPase activity are Type IIB. I = Type I fiber. a = Type IIA fiber. b = Type IIB fiber.*

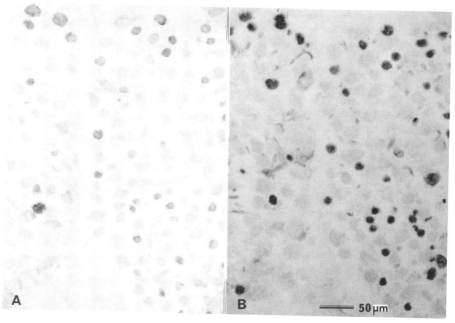

Figure 8-4. *Serial sections of orbital layer of extraocular muscle. A: anti-ALD. B: AT-Pase at pH 4.4. Fibers stained with anti-ALD correspond to fibers with acid-stable AT-Pase activity.*

that has been used to identify single tonic fibers in extraocular muscles and analyze their ultrastructural characteristics (Bach-y-Rita, Lennerstrach, Alvarado, Nichols, and McHolm, 1977). In human extraocular muscles, the fibers labeled by anti-ALD have multiple end-plates and therefore probably correspond to slow tonic fibers (Pierobon, Sartore, Vitadello and Schiaffino, 1980). Nothing is known about the physiological properties of multiply innervated fibers in the laryngeal muscle, but on the basis of the previous observations, the multiply innervated fibers with acid-stable ATPase activity in the TA are probably slow twitch fibers.

The muscle fibers of phasic active motoneurons usually contract and relax rapidly. Type I fibers are easily distinguishable from Type II fibers by their strong histochemical reaction for myosin ATPase. This was also true of the TA. In contrast, two major subgroups of fast twitch fibers, IIA and IIB fibers, can usually be distinguished histochemically by differences in the pH-stability of their ATPase activity, but this was not so in the TA: subgroups of Type II fibers could not be distinguished. Gradual inactivation of Type II fiber ATPase activity at pH 4.4-4.65 has been noted in human extraocular muscles (Nunomura, Hizawa, Li, and Sano, 1984). Because the contraction time of the TA in cats (15 to 21ms) is fast compared with the contraction times of mammalian limb muscles (Gauthier and Padykula, 1966), the multiply innervated fibers with alkali-stable myosin ATPase activity are expected to be fast fibers. Possibly the multiply innervated Type II

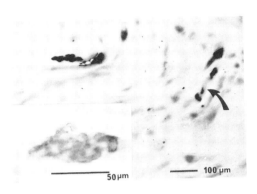

Figure 8-5. *TA. Multiply innervated fiber (arrowhead) is noted in this longitudinally cut fiber and the morphology of these end-plates is similar to en plaque neuromuscular junction (inset): AchE.*

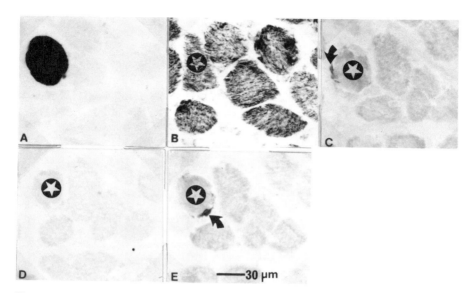

Figure 8-6. *Serial sections of TA. A: ATPase at pH 4.35. B: NADH-TR. C,D,E: AchE. Multiply innervated fiber (asterisk) with acid-stable ATPase activity is seen. C-E=100 μm.*

fibers of laryngeal muscles correspond to the multiply innervated twitch fibers of the external eye muscles in cats (Bendiksen, et al., 1981).

Most TA fibers with alkali-stable ATPase activity were rich in glycolytic enzymes and moderately rich in enzymes of aerobic oxidative metabolism. This indicates that most of the muscle fibers in the human TA should be metabolically resistant to fatigue during prolonged activity.

Comparative studies on various mammals have indicated a relation between the rate of breathing and the capacity for aerobic oxidation, as represented by the activity of succinic dehydrogenase (SDH) in fibers of the diaphragm (Gauthier and Padykula, 1966; Green, Reichmann and Pette, 1984). The enzyme pattern of energy metabolism seems to be related to the normal amount and type of activity of the muscle. These findings suggest that the characteristics of TA fibers in energy metabolism may reflect adaptation to both rapid contraction times and fatigue resistance.

Type IIA and IIB fibers in humans represent populations with a large scatter and overlap of aerobic oxidative capacities (Reichmann and Pette, 1982). Quantitative analyses of muscles of different species have shown that the contents of mitochondrial and cytosolic enzymes of individual fibers vary over wide ranges in each of the ATPase-based fiber types (I, IIA, IIB) (Lowry, Kimmey, Felder, et al., 1978). The variability of metabolic profiles, myosin compositions, and modes of innervation of TA fibers may thus be a reflection of the fact that motor units cannot be rigidly classified into three types, but that they form a continuous spectrum with re-

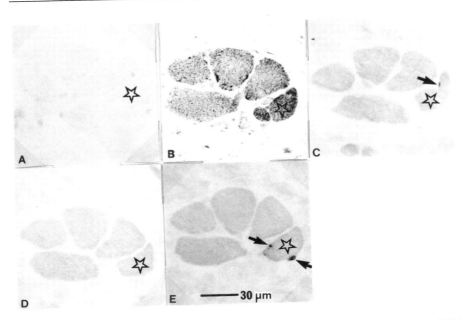

Figure 8-7. *Serial sections of thyroarytenoid muscle. A: ATPase at pH 4.35. B: NADH-TR. C,D,E: AchE. Multiply innervated fiber (asterisk) with acid-labile ATPase activity is seen. C-E = 300 μm.*

gard to readiness for recruitment (Navarrete and Vrbova, 1983). Consistent with this idea, the threshold of a motoneuron is inversely related to its size (i.e., the smallest neurons are most readily excited), and there is no indication that the sizes of the alpha motoneurons fall into three distinct groups (Henneman, Somjen, and Carpenter, 1965; Henneman, Clamann, Gil-

lies, and Skinner, 1984).

The different patterns of glottic profiles in diverse vocal activities can be achieved only by selective muscular contraction. Neurophysiological studies are required to determine how the motor units of the TA are related to diversified muscular activity according to differences in their physiological activities.

REFERENCES

Bach-y-Rita, P., and Ito, F. (1966). In vivo studies on fast and slow muscle fibers in cat extraocular muscles. *J Gen Physiol, 49,* 1177–1198.

Bach-y-Rita, P., Lennerstrand, G., Alvarado, J., Nichols, K., and Mcholm, G. (1977). Extraocular muscle fibers: Ultrastructural identification of iontophoretically labeled fibers contracting in response to succinylcholine. *Invert Ophthalmol Visual Sci, 16,* 561–564.

Bendiksen, F.S., Dahl, H.A., and Tei, E. (1981). Innervation pattern of different types of muscle fibers in human thyroarytenoid muscle. *Acta Otolaryngol, 91,* 391–397.

Dietert, S.E. (1965). The demonstration of different types of muscle fibers in human extraocular muscle by electron microscopy and cholinesterase staining. *Invest Ophthalmol, 4,* 51.

Dubuwitz, V., and Brooke, M.H. (1973). *Muscle biopsy: A modern approach.* London: Sanders.

Garnett, R.A.F., O'Donovan, M.J., Stephens, J.A., and Taylor, A. (1978). Motor unit organization of human medial gastrocnemius. *J Physiol, 287,* 33–43.

Gauthier, G.F., and Padykula, H.A. (1966). Cytological studies of fiber types in skeletal muscle. A comparative study of the mammalian diaphragm. *J Cell Biol, 28,* 333–354.

Ginsborg, B.L. (1960). Some properties of avian skeletal muscle fibers with multiple neuromuscular junctions. *J Physiol, 154,* 581–598.

Green, H.J., Reichmann, H., and Pette, D. (1984). Inter- and intraspecies comparisons of fiber type distribution and of succinate dehydrogenase activity in Type I, IIA, and IIB fibers of mammalian diaphragms. *Histochemie, 81,* 67–73.

Henneman, E., Clamann, H.P., Gillies, J.D., and Skinner, R.D. (1974). Rank order of motoneurons within a pool: law of combination. *J Neurophysiol, 37,* 1338–1349.

Henneman, E., Somjen, G., and Carpenter, D.O. (1965). Functional significance of cell size in spinal motoneurons. *J Neurophysiol, 28,* 560–580.

Hess, A. (1970). Vertebrate slow muscle fibers. *Physiol Rev, 50,* 40–62.

Hess, A., and Pilar, G. (1963). Slow fibers in the extraocular muscle of the cat. *J Physiol, 169,* 780–798.

Hsu, S.M., Rainel, L., and Fanger, H. (1981). Use of avidin-biotin-peroxidase techniques: A comparison between ABC and unlabelled antibody (PAP) procedure. *J Histochem Cytochem, 29,* 577–581.

Koelle, G.B., Friendenwald, J.S. (1966). Comparison of the gold-thiocholine and gold-thiolacetic acid methods for the histochemical localization of acetyicholinesterase and cholinesterase. *J Histochem Cytochem, 14,* 443–454.

Lowery, C.V., Kimmey, J.S., Felder, S., et al. (1978). Enzyme patterns in single human muscle fibers. *J Biol Chem, 253,* 8269–8277.

Matyrushkin, D.P. (1961). Phasic and tonic neuromotor units in the oculomotor apparatus of the rabbit. *Sechenov Physiol J USSR, 46,* 65.

Meijer, A.E. (1968). Improved histochemical methods for demonstration of the activity of alpha-glucan phosphorylase. I. The use of glycosyl acceptor dextran. *Histochemie, 12,* 144–151.

Morales, J., Rama, J., and Gayoso, M. (1980). Some aspects of the nerve endings and synapses in the vocalis muscle. *J Laryngol Otol, 94,* 1047–1063.

Mortensson, A., and Skoglund, C.R. (1964). Contraction properties of intrinsic laryngeal muscle. *Acta Physiol Scand, 60,* 318–336.

Navarrete, R., and Vrbova, G. (1983). Changes of activity patterns in slow and fast muscles during postnatal development. *Dev Brain Res, 8,* 11–19.

Nunomura, S., Hizawa, K., Li, K., and Sano, T. (1984). A histochemical study on fiber types in human extraocular muscle. *Biomedical Res, 5,* 295–302.

Pierobon, B.S., Sartore, S., Vitadello, M., and Schiaffino, S. (1980). "Slow" myosins in vertebrate skeletal muscle. An immunofluorescence study. *J Cell Biol, 85,* 672–681.

Pierobon, B.S., Torresan, S., Sartore, G.B., Moschini, G., Schiaffino, S. (1979). Immunohistochemical identification of slow tonic fibers in human extrinsic eye muscles. *Invest Ophthalmol Visual Sci, 18,* 303–306.

Reichmann, H., and Pette, D. (1982). A comparative microphotometric study of succinate dehydrogenase activity levels in Type I, IIA, IIB fibers of mammalian and human muscles. *Histochemie, 74,* 27–41.

Rosenfield, D.B., Miller, R.H., Sessions, R.B., and Patten, B.M. (1982). Morphologic and histochemical characteristics of laryngeal muscle. *Arch Otolaryngol, 108,* 662–666.

Walton, J.N., and Bardner-Nedwin, D. (1974). Progressive muscular dystrophy and the myotonic disorders. In J.N. Walton (Ed.), *Disorders of Voluntary Muscle* (3rd ed.) (pp. 561–613), Edinburgh: Churchill Livingstone.

CHAPTER 9

Mechanical Properties of the Intrinsic Laryngeal Muscles and Biomechanics of the Glottis in Dogs

Fumihiko SATO
and Yasuo HISA

I t is well known that glottic movements are regulated by complex and coordinated activities of the laryngeal muscles during swallowing, coughing, phonation, and respiration.

We previously reported that vocal fold position depended on the frequency of electrical stimulations applied to the laryngeal nerves (Sato, Yanohara, Takenouchi, Suzuki, Hisa, and Hiuga, 1982). When both recurrent laryngeal nerves were stimulated at 0.1 ms, 1 volt, at 20 to 25 Hz, the vocal folds abducted. As the stimulation frequency was increased beyond 25 Hz, the vocal folds adducted. When the external branch of the superior laryngeal nerve was bilaterally stimulated at 10 to 20 Hz, the vocal folds flicked simultane-

ously with each stimulus. When the frequency was increased to 20 to 30 Hz, the vocal folds were adducted and elongated. This raised the question as to what determined this response: nerve fibers, motor end plates, or muscle fibers. Further investigation revealed that the fibers of each muscle were the determining elements.

In this paper, we studied the relationship between contraction time, fusion frequency, and glottic configuration caused by contraction of individual laryngeal muscles.

Studies of contraction properties of intrinsic laryngeal muscles have usually used cats, rather than dogs, as experimental animals (Hast, 1964; Martensson and

Skoglund, 1964; Hast, 1966; 1967; 1969). Dogs were used in this study.

METHODS

Contraction Properties of Intrinsic Laryngeal Muscles

Treatment of Larynx

Eight hybrid mature dogs each weighing 10 to 13 Kg were used. Anesthesia was induced with ketamine hydrochloride injected intramuscularly, and maintained with intravenous thiopental sodium.

The laryngeal muscles were exposed through a median cervical skin incision. A displacement tension transducer (F-D transducer) was attached to one end of each muscle while the other end was fixed (Figure 9-1). Tension was measured in each intrinsic laryngeal muscle during isometric contraction.

The Cricothyroid Muscle (CT)

The cricoid cartilage was divided at the point of insertion of the CT. It was connected to the F-D transducer by means of a plastic suture fixed to a metal stand. The thyroid cartilage was similarly fixed.

The Thyroarytenoid Muscle (TA)

Following laryngofissure, the thyroid cartilage was sectioned at the attachment of the TA and connected to a transducer. Medical

adhesive Aronalpha[R] was instilled into the cricoarytenoid joint to fix the arytenoid cartilage.

The Posterior Cricoarytenoid Muscle (PCA)

In order to expose the PCA, the inferior pharyngeal constrictor and the inferior horn of the thyroid cartilage were removed. The arytenoid cartilage was detached from the cricoid cartilage at the cricoarytenoid joint. The thyroarytenoid, lateral cricoarytenoid, and arytenoid muscles were separated from the arytenoid cartilage. The arytenoid cartilage was then connected to the F-D transducer with a plastic suture.

The Lateral Cricoarytenoid Muscle (LCA)

The LCA was exposed by the same approach used for the PCA. All muscles other than the LCA were removed from the arytenoid cartilage, and it was connected to the transducer. This procedure required very careful surgical technique because the LCA is a small muscle.

Experimental Equipment and Methods

The transducer system consisted of a Nihon Kode F-D Pick-Up SB-1T connected to a RP-5 preamplifier and an oscilloscope VC 7. The contraction curve of each intrinsic laryngeal muscle was photographed from the screen of the oscilloscope in most cases. In others, it was recorded

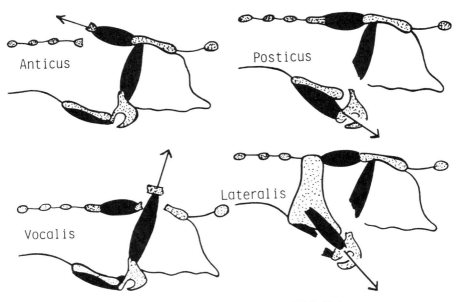

Figure 9-1. *Direction of pull toward F-D Pick-up.*

by means of a recticorder RJG-3014.

Electrical stimulation of 0.1 ms 1 volt rectangular waves was delivered to each intrinsic laryngeal muscle with a platinum bipolar electrode connected to a Nihon Koden stimulator MSE-3R, permitting measurement of contraction time and fusion frequency from a twitch and tetanus contraction curve.

To prevent dryness and fall in tissue temperature, a warm physiological saline solution was continuously applied to the tissues, maintaining the temperature at 37 to 38°C. Stimulation time was limited to 2 s with a 5 s resting interval between each stimulus to prevent muscular fatigue. After an initial tension of 3 to 5 g was applied, stimulation was started.

Morphology and Dynamics of the Glottis Due to Each Intrinsic Laryngeal Muscle Contraction

The experimental design was essentially the same as that used in determining the contraction properties. Briefly, the stimulus was delivered directly to the recurrent nerve at a point about 2 cm from the muscle after removing all other branches except the one supplying the muscle. The distance between the vocal processes and the length of the glottis were determined from photographs of the glottis. Glottic pressure was determined by means of a cylinder-type pressure receptor and a transducer. Finally, the tension at the vocal process during adduction and abduction was determined by an F-D Pick-Up. In this series, we observed how changes in these parameters were affected by stimulus frequency.

RESULTS

Contraction Properties of Intrinsic Laryngeal Muscles

Table 9-1 summarizes the contraction properties of each intrinsic laryngeal muscle. Each contraction time was recorded as a mean whole number value. The most frequent fusion frequency was also recorded. The intrinsic laryngeal muscles were generally rapid or fast muscles compared to skeletal muscles. The TA was the most rapid, followed by the LCA and the PCA. On the other hand, the fusion frequency was 95 Hz for the TA, 90 Hz for the LCA, 45 Hz for the PCA, and 40 Hz for the CT. Thus, the fusion frequency was higher in those muscles with the fastest contraction times (Sato and Ogura, 1978). This was most obvious in the TA.

Contraction Properties as They Relate to Morphology and Glottal Dynamics

The CT (Figure 9-2): Vocal fold elongation was maximum at 40 to 45 Hz and the glottal width was reduced. Coincidental with these changes, the glottic pressure and the adduction tension in the horizontal plane were maximum. Further changes were not observed with stimulation at higher frequencies. On the other hand, the fusion frequency of this muscle was 40 Hz, and the glottic pressure and adduction tension was also maximum at this point. The stimulation frequency at which the maximum morphologic change of the glottis occurred corresponded to the fusion frequency. This indicates that glottic configuration was determined by contraction of the muscle itself, and not by other structures such as the ligament.

The PCA (Figure 9-3): At 30 to 40 Hz, the vocal fold was maximally abducted, and showed maximum tension. Below this frequency the vocal fold oscillated at the same frequency as that of the stimulus. Thus, the fusion frequency of 45 Hz and the stimulation frequency for maximum abduction and tension were nearly identical. The properties of the PCA were, therefore, similar to those of the CT.

The TA (Figure 9-4): Glottic pressure and vocal fold length was maximum at 95 to 100 Hz. Fusion frequency was also 95 Hz, corresponding to the frequency at which glottic pressure was maximum and vocal fold length minimum. However, this frequency did not correspond to that which produced minimum glottic width or maximum tension on adduction. The inter-glottic distance was shortest at 60 Hz and the tension on adduction in the horizontal plane was maximum at 80 Hz. The differences exhibited by this muscle are due to the anatomical configuration, which kept the vocal process from sliding forward and adducting.

The LCA (Figure 9-5): Fusion frequency of the muscle was 90 Hz. The glottis completely closed at 60 Hz, and the tension on adduction

TABLE 9-1.
Contraction Properties in Canine Intrinsic Laryngeal Muscles

	CT	TA	PCA	LCA
Contraction time	38 msec	14 msec	42 msec	21 msec
Half-relaxation time	31.7 msec	16 msec	37.2 msec	22.5 msec
Tetanus: twitch tension ratio	4.5	7.1	3.8	6.8
Fusion frequency	40 Hz	95 Hz	45 Hz	90 Hz

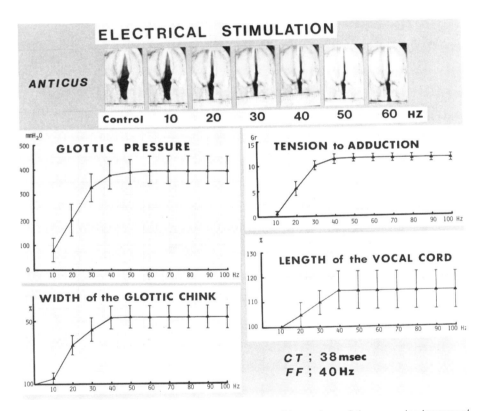

Figure 9-2. *Electrical stimulation to both external branches of the superior laryngeal nerves. All results were constant at 35 to 40 Hz, corresponding to the fusion frequency.*

101

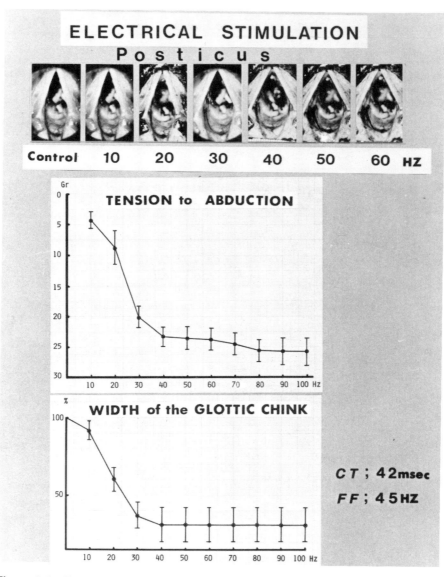

Figure 9-3. *Electrical stimulation to the bilateral PCA branch. Characteristics of the determination method prevented determination of glottic closure pressure. However, in both graphs at 40 to 45 Hz the glottis opened at maximum tension and width. No change occurred at increased frequency. The fusion frequency was 45 Hz.*

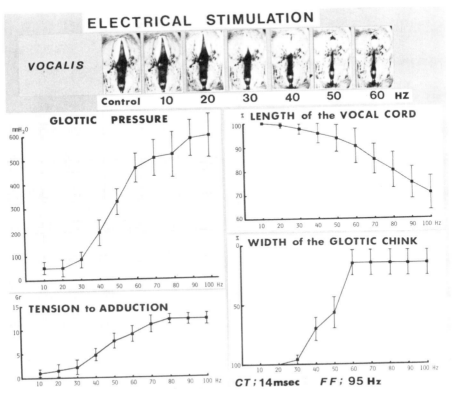

Figure 9-4. *Electrical stimulation of nerve branches to both TAs. Fusion frequency was 95 Hz. Glottic closure tension and width were restricted by anatomical factors at 60 to 70 Hz. At higher frequencies, sphincteric action was increased.*

gradually increased from 40 Hz to a maximum at 80 to 90 Hz. This powerful glottic closure may be related to the compensatory adduction of the healthy vocal fold often seen in unilateral recurrent nerve paralysis.

The transverse arytenoid muscle (Figure 9-6): It was difficult to determine the contraction properties of this muscle. However, from the results of glottic pressure, adduction tension, and inter-glottic distance, the fusion frequency was inferred to be 75 Hz, and the

properties of the muscle itself were inferred to be similar to the TA and the LCA.

DISCUSSION

Examination of the contraction properties of the intrinsic laryngeal muscles as they relate to movements of the anatomical structures such as the cricoarytenoid joint and arytenoid cartilage produced several interesting observations. Glottic dynamics were clearly

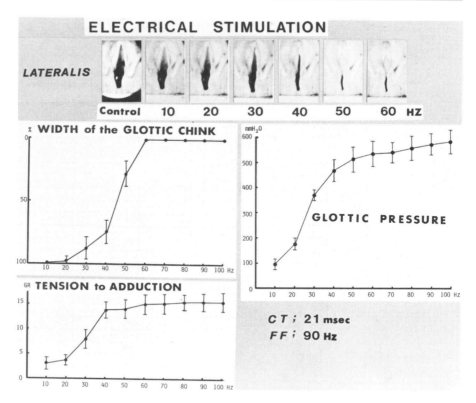

Figure 9-5. *Electrical stimulation to nerve branch to each LCA. As with the TA at 60 Hz, the width of the glottis was zero, and at 85 to 95 Hz, glottic closure tension was maximum. Stimulation frequency at which glottic closure tension and pressure were maximum corresponded to the fusion frequency. However, inter-glottic distance was zero at 60 Hz, the added power probably being due to compensatory adduction.*

affected by the physical properties of the intrinsic laryngeal muscles. However, glottic movements could not be accounted for solely on the basis of the physical properties of individual laryngeal muscles. Glottic configuration is also influenced by the properties of the motor nerves and by physical features of laryngeal anatomy. In this investigation, stimulation was applied to the motor nerve at a short distance from the muscle to determine the type of glottic move-

ment. For this reason, results may have been affected by properties of the nerve itself, such as differences in sensitivity to the stimulus frequency or differences in conduction velocity. Results were similar when the muscle was stimulated directly and when its motor nerve was stimulated. Thus, the relationship between glottic movement, muscle properties and mechanical effects of individual muscle contraction have been clarified by this experiment. The

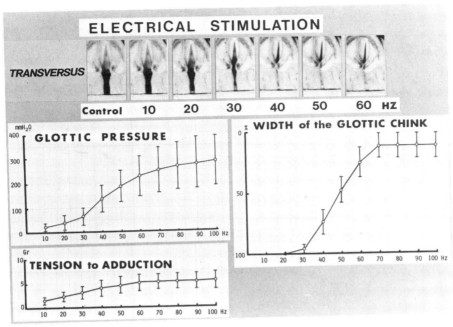

Figure 9-6. *Electrical stimulation to both branches supplying the arytenoid muscle. From the results it was inferred that the fusion frequency of the muscle itself was more than 70 Hz.*

anatomical factors that can restrict or influence glottic movement are listed in Table 9-2. Most of the restriction is caused by ligaments, the "membrane frame," and the elastic recoil, but the morphology of the cricoid and arytenoid cartilages and of the cricoarytenoid joint also influence glottic configuration.

In conclusion, this study demonstrates the complex dynamic inter-

TABLE 9.2
Anatomical Structures Affecting Glottic Movement

Conus elasticus
Cricothyroid membrane
Quadrangular membrane
Posterior cricoarytenoid ligament
Cricoarytenoid capsule
Vocal ligament
Thyrohyoid ligament
Cricoarytenoid joint
Shape of the cricoid and arytenoid cartilage

play of the intrinsic laryngeal muscles and the anatomical structures to which they are attached. The LCA and the TA influence the passage of air by a type of glottic sphincteric action. The LCA was shown to provide the power necessary for compensatory adduction in unilateral recurrent laryngeal nerve paralysis. Furthermore, the data suggest that spastic dysphonia might be treated by selective resection of the nerve branch to the LCA or the TA, rather than resecting the entire recurrent laryngeal nerve.

These findings should help clarify some of the basic considerations in studying the complex glottic movements created by contraction of the intrinsic laryngeal muscles.

REFERENCES

Hast, M.H. (1964). Chronaxie of the vocal folds of the dog. *Ann Otol, 73*, 305–311.

Hast, M.H. (1966). Mechanical properties of the cricothyroid muscle. *Laryngoscope, 76*, 537–548.

Hast, M.H. (1967). Mechanical properties of the vocal fold muscle. *Pract Otol Rhinol Laryngol 29*, 53–56.

Hast, M.H. (1969). The primate larynx: A comparative physiological study of intrinsic muscles. *Acta Otolaryngol, 67*, 84–92.

Mårtensson, A., and Skoglund, C.R. (1964). Contraction properties of intrinsic laryngeal muscles. *Acta Physiol Scand, 60*, 318–336.

Sato, F., Yanohara, K., Takenouchi, S., Suzuki, Y., Hisa, Y., and Hiuga, M. (1982). Effect of contraction of each intrinsic laryngeal muscle on shape and biomechanics of glottis. *J Jpn Bronchoesophagol Soc, 33*, 302–308.

CHAPTER 10

A Histochemical Study of Denervated Intrinsic Laryngeal Muscle

Sei-ichi RYU

Changes occurring in the muscles of the extremities after denervation have been investigated by the usual histopathological (Broeckaert, 1904; Grabower, 1909) and histochemical techniques (Bajusz, 1964; Hogenhuis and Engel, 1965; Engel, Brooke, and Nelson, 1966; Karpati and Engel, 1968; Rosenfield, Miller, Sessions, and Patten, 1982; Sahgal and Hast, 1974; Warmolts, 1981). However, there have been relatively few studies of recurrent laryngeal nerve paralysis. In this study, recurrent nerve paralysis was produced experimentally and the histochemical changes were investigated in the fibers of four intrinsic laryngeal muscles. Results and clinical implications of the findings are discussed.

HISTOCHEMICAL ACTIVITY IN NORMAL LARYNGEAL MUSCLES

The normal histochemical activity in the canine laryngeal muscles has been reported (Ryu, 1982). The staining pattern of the laryngeal muscles generally fell into two types. Type I muscle fiber showed low activity for ATPase, and phosphorylase, but high activity for nicotine amidadenin dinucleotic dehydrogenase (NADH) and succinic dehydrogenase (SDH). In contrast, Type II muscle fiber exhibited high activity for ATPase and phosphorylase, and low activity for NADH and SDH (Table 10-1).

The distribution of the two types of muscle fibers differed for each intrinsic laryngeal muscle. The percentage of Type I muscle fibers to the whole muscle in the interarytenoid (IA), lateral cricoarytenoid (LCA), thyroarytenoid (TA), and posterior cricoarytenoid muscle (PCA) was 10, 12, 13, and 40 percent, respectively (Ryu, 1982). Figure 10-1 shows some photomicrographs illustrating these differences.

The IAs and LCAs have a uniform distribution pattern throughout the muscle. In the TA, the distribution of the two muscle fiber types showed a large variation in distribution. Type I muscle fibers were primarily situated in the medial part of the muscle, gradually decreasing and nearly disappearing in the lateral part. It was in the PCA that Type II muscle fibers were most evident.

MATERIALS AND METHODS

Adult dogs weighing about 10 Kg were anesthesized with ketamine by intramuscular injection. The neck was opened at the midline. The recurrent nerve on one side was carefully exposed and was traumatized near the thyroid gland by one of the following three methods:

1. In Group 1, a 1 cm segment of the recurrent nerve was removed surgically.
2. In Group 2, the nerve was merely sectioned.
3. In Group 3, the nerves were traumatically crushed with hemostatic forceps.

Complete immobility of the vocal fold by direct laryngoscopy was used to confirm the paralysis.

TABLE 10.1
Histochemical Activity of Muscle Fiber

Staining	Muscle Fiber Type	
	Type I	Type II
ATPhase (pH 9.4)	low	high
Phosphorylase	low	high
NADH	high	low
SDH	high	low

A

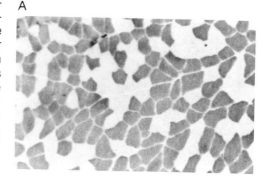

B

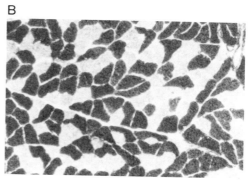

Figure 10-1. *Enzyme activities of normal laryngeal muscles. A: Cricothyroid muscle: stained with ATPase pH 9.4. Dark stained muscle fibers are Type II. Light (red in color) stained muscle fibers are Type I. B: PCA: stained with ATPase pH 9.4. The proportion of Type I muscle fibers within the entire muscle is similar to the pattern in the cricothyroid. C: PCA: stained with phosphorylase. Dark (blue stained) muscle fibers are Type II, of high activity, and the red- stained fibers are Type I fibers of low activity. D: PCA: stained with NADH. Dark stained muscle fibers*

(continued page 109)

Each month after operation, two animals of each group were sacrificed for histochemical studies of the laryngeal muscles. Vocal fold paralysis was verified before the animal was killed. Four intrinsic laryngeal muscles, namely, the TA, PCA, LCA, and IA were bilaterally removed. The muscles were trimmed and frozen in liquid acetone dry ice. The specimens were then fixed on a metal stage and serial cross sections were cut by cryostat.

Histochemical studies of the sections were performed by staining for the presence of myofibrillar ATPase (pH 9.4) according to Padykula and Hermann (1955); phosphorylase according to Takenouchi and Kuriaki (1955); reduced NADH according to Barka and Anderson (1963); and SDH according to Nachales et al. (1957). Hematoxylin-eosin staining was also done for routine histopathological examination.

Enzyme activity in the fibers of the four intrinsic laryngeal muscles were studied in relation to (1) percentage of Type I fibers to the whole muscle; (2) distribution pattern of Type I and Type II muscle fibers; (3) mobility, if present, of the vocal fold; and (4) macroscopic and microscopic muscle atrophy.

RESULTS

Group 1

Mobility of Vocal Folds

There were no signs of recovery of vocal fold mobility observed at any stage after partial removal of the nerve.

C

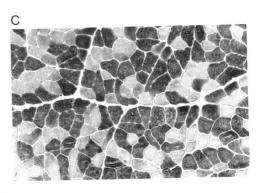

D

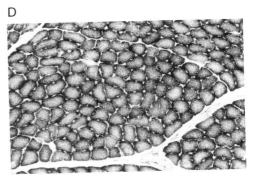

E

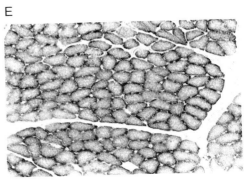

Figure 10-1 (*continued*):

are Type I and light stained muscle fibers are Type II. E: PCA: stained with SDH. Dark stained muscle fibers are Type I and light stained muscle fibers are Type II fibers. F: LCA: stained with ATPase pH 9.4. Type II muscle fiber is dominant and distributed like a "checkerboard." G: TA: stained with ATPase pH 9.4. Type II muscle fiber is dominant in the peripheral part in the left and Type I muscle fiber demonstrates a
(*continued page 110*)

Macrographic Observation

Muscular atrophy gradually increased each month after resection.

Enzyme Activity

ATPase activity in both Type I and Type II muscle fibers did not decrease even in the sixth month after nerve resection (Figure 10-2A). Phosphorylase activity started decreasing one month after resection and was totally absent by the third month (Figure 10-2B). The activity of NADH and SDH decreased gradually over the course of the first month (Figure 10-2C). The degree of decreased SDH activity was more marked than that of NADH activity. We observed no differences in the alteration of enzyme activity in the four intrinsic laryngeal muscles studied.

Morphological Change

Type I muscle fibers generally atrophied more slowly than Type II. They even appeared to enlarge in the first three months after resection (Figure 10-2D). Type II muscle fibers began to atrophy in the second month, and the degree of atrophy increased in subsequent months (Figure 10-2D). Differences in the diameter of Type I and Type II muscle fibers were observed also with hema-toxylin-eosin staining (Figure 10-2E).

Distribution Ratio of Type I and Type II Muscle Fibers

Neither distribution pattern nor distribution ratio were observed to

F

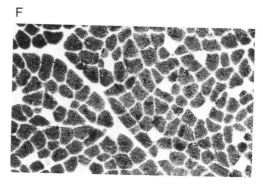

G

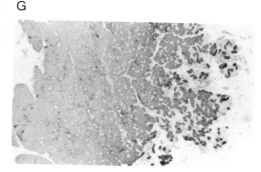

H

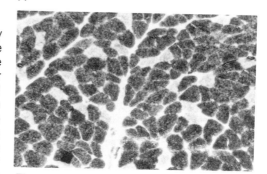

Figure 10-1 (*continued*):

gradual increase from the periphery to the inner portion on the right. H: IA: stained with ATPase pH 9.4. Shows similar results with that of the LCA. Type II muscle fibers are dominant and distributed like a patchwork quilt.

change in any of the muscles except those that appeared to be reinnervated.

Reinnervation

Although complete reinnervation was not seen in any of the animals, partial reinnervation was observed in the fifth month or later (Figure 10-2F). In some instances, groupings of specific muscle fibers formed in several muscle bundles.

Groups 2 and 3

Mobility of the Vocal Fold

The mobility of the vocal fold did not improve during the experimental period.

Morphological Changes

Atrophy in Type II muscle fibers occasionally occurred in Group 2 after the second month, but no clear atrophy was observed in Group 3. The degree of atrophy varied for the four muscles studied. For example, even when both the LCA and the TA were atrophic, the IA was not (Figure 10-3). The morphological changes observed in Type I muscle fibers of Groups 2 and 3 were similar to the findings in Group I. In all three cases the fibers tended to enlarge.

Enzyme Activity

No change in ATPase activity was noted in either group. In selected examples, NADH and SDH activity was decreased, but the lower activity levels did not appear to correlate with the length

A

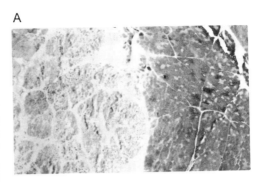

B

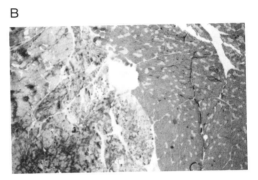

Figure 10-2. *Enzyme activities after recurrent nerve was resected. A: Fifth month after resection; the LCA stained with ATPase. The experimental side is on the left and the control side is on the right. Enzyme activity was observed in the experimental side and Type I muscle fiber was dominant. B: Fifth month after resection; the LCA stained with phosphorylase. The experimental side is on the left and the control side is on the right. No enzyme activity was ob-*

(continued page 112)

of time post surgery. There were no histochemical changes observed in Group 3.

Reinnervation

Reinnervation was not observed in Group 3 at any time. In contrast, groupings in some specific muscle fibers were observed in Group 2 as early as one month following the nerve resection. When grouping was observed, it generally occurred in all the muscles at nearly the same time.

Table 10-2 summarizes the changes in enzyme activity associated with the three types of trauma.

DISCUSSION

In this experiment, a clinically important condition was simulated by three types of trauma applied to the recurrent laryngeal nerve (section, partial resection, and crushing). The muscles were then studied histochemically to observe changes occurring in the paralyzed muscles. The most severe trauma to the nerve appeared to be resection. The least traumatic was crushing.

From the general pathological point of view, denervated muscle fibers atrophy first and simultaneously lose their stripes. The muscle plasma becomes granular, vacuoles appear inside the plasma, and the muscle becomes fragmented. Finally, histiocytic myophagia ensues, and the muscle fiber is replaced by connective tissue (Seddon, 1975).

In Group 1, where the nerve was partially removed, there was theo-

C

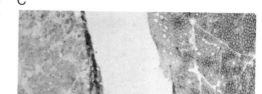

D

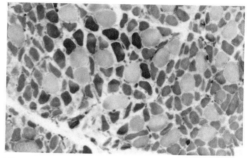

Figure 10-2 (*continued*):

served. C: Third month after resection; the LCA stained with SDH. The experimental side is on the left, the normal side is on the right. SDH activity decreased and NADH showed almost identical activity. D: Second month after resection; the LCA stained with ATPase. Hypertrophied Type I muscle fibers and atrophied

(*continued page 113*)

retically little possibility of reinnervation, and the muscle fibers should have gone through the typical processes of denervation. Most of the enzyme activity was gradually lowered, with some observable differences between the enzymes studied. The decrease of activity was most marked with phosphorylase, followed by NADH, SDH, and ATPase, in that order. The phosphorylase activity began to drop in the first month and within three months was nearly absent. In the crushed specimens, phosphorylase activity did not change. Therefore, the third month was interpreted as being the critical point in muscle function and atrophy. Perhaps atrophy could be avoided if reinnervation occurred before the third month.

The activities of oxidative enzymes such as NADH and SDH were reduced in both the resected and sectioned group. Many other investigators have reported that the stronger the initial activity, the greater the eventual loss (Nachimias and Padykula, 1964; Romanual, 1965; Smith, 1965; Engel et al., 1966; Wuerker and Bodley, 1973). The IA, even in Group 1, did not always show reduced oxidative enzymes compared to the contralateral control side. This is consistent with the bilateral innervation of this muscle.

Because ATPase activity was the least likely to be lost, muscle fibers could be classified even when other enzyme activity was absent or decreased. Swelling of Type I muscle fibers always occurred in Group 1 and occasionally in Group 2. By contrast, Type II fibers showed steady atrophy and decreased diameters. These

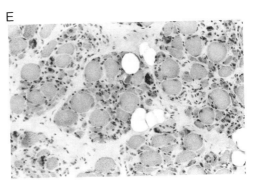

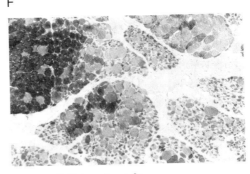

Figure 10-2 (*continued*):

Type II muscle fibers where observed. E: Third month after resection; the LCA stained with hematoxylin-eosin, illustrates fiber size changes. F: Fifth month after resection; the LCA stained with phosphorylase. Enzyme activity was recovered at the time of partial reinnervation.

changes almost all occurred within three months. Peak swelling of Type I muscle fibers reportedly occurred around three or four weeks post denervation in rats (Bajusz, 1964; Engel et al., 1966; Karpati and Engel, 1968). Nearly identical results were observed in dogs in the current experiment.

In the crush-injury group, changes in all enzyme activities seldom occurred, nor was there any atrophy. Crushing may not affect function at the muscle cell level, or perhaps there is immediate onset of reinnervation. It is puzzling why these histological changes do not result in recovery of vocal fold movement.

Grouping, as used here, means clustering of muscle fibers of the same type after reinnervation, in contrast to normal muscle in which the two types of fibers are evenly scattered. This grouping was most often observed in Group 2, and least often in Group 1. When reinnervation was successful, it occurred in all laryngeal muscles at the same time. It appears that the cut end of the recurrent nerve in Group 2 is in such close proximity to the muscle that reinnervation of the muscle fibers occurs quickly, but through misdirection. In Group 1, the cut ends are sufficiently distant, about 1 cm apart, to prevent reinnervation. In Group 3, by contrast, there was no grouping. It may be assumed that the nerve sheath was not sectioned in this group, so that misdirection of the innervating fibers was less likely to occur.

We believe that these findings of misdirection add further clarification to the paradoxical movement sometimes observed after section of the recurrent laryngeal nerve.

A
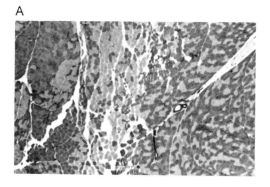

B
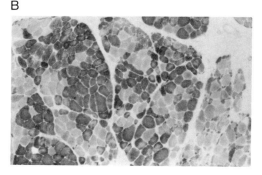

Figure 10-3. *Enzyme activity after the recurrent nerve was dissected. A: Sixth month after dissection; the PCA stained with ATPase. The experimental side is on the left and the normal side is on the right. Type I and II fibers are grouped on the experimental side. B: Sixth month after dissection; the LCA stained with phosphorylase. Grouping patterns were simi-*

(continued page 115)

Nerves occasionally regenerated, with recovery of all enzyme activities in the regional muscles. However, the reinnervated muscle fibers varied considerably in size. These differences may explain the occasional incomplete recovery of muscle contractibility.

Because "fiber type grouping" has also been observed in the human PCA, some investigators consider this grouping to be evidence of weakness, and the reason for abduction weakness sometimes observed in loud-speaking persons (Gunn, 1972; Gunn, 1973; Edstrom, Linquist, and Martensson, 1974; Malmgren, 1981).

Without exception, the reinnervation varied with the degree of damage to the nerve. There was a discrepancy between the vocal fold mobility and enyzme activity, particularly in Group 3.

There is a difference in the way that Type I and Type II muscle fibers undergo atrophy after nerve section. Type I fibers tend to temporarily enlarge for one or two months immediately after denervation, whereas Type II fibers atrophy steadily from the beginning. This is consistent with reports of differences in fiber size as observed by conventional hematoxylin-eosin staining.

The difference in the course of atrophy between Type I and Type II fibers accounts, in part, for the degree of atrophy that can be observed grossly in a given muscle. In addition, the duration of denervation contributes to the degree of observable atrophy. It is assumed that only the recovery of Type I muscle fiber is dependent upon the reinnervation period.

Prior to the current study, there

C
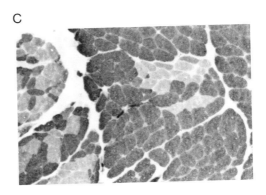

D
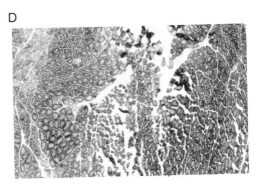

Figure 10-3 (*continued*):

lar to those seen in the PCA. C: Sixth month after dissection; the TA stained with ATPase. Grouping was similar to that seen in the PCA and the LCA. D: Sixth month after dissection; the IA stained with NADH. The experimental side is on the left and the control side is on the right. Lowered activity was not observed in either side.

TABLE 10-2.
The Change of Enzyme Activity in the Muscle Fiber Due to Trauma

Group	Atrophy	ATPhase	Phosphorylase	NADH & SDH
1	Marked (Type I, hypertrophied; Type II, atrophied)	Almost no change	Disappeared within three months	Slightly decreased
2	Slight ~ moderate	No change	No change or decreased	No change or slightly decreased
3	None ~ slight	No change	No change or slightly decreased	No change

was little information on which of the intrinsic laryngeal muscles atrophies fastest after denervation. Available studies are not in agreement (Lee, 1965; Izuka, 1966; Hall-Craggs, 1968; Nagashima, 1970). From the current study on dogs, the PCA showed the least atrophy in the early stages because of its rich supply of Type I muscle fibers. In contrast, the TA and the LCA seemed to atrophy most rapidly because of the predominance of Type II fibers.

Although there are many differences between the anatomy of dogs and humans, the current study may add further evidence to those reports now available on human recurrent nerve paralysis. When paralysis occurs in the human larynx, histochemical studies suggest that the TA, LCA, and IA undergo early atrophy because of their high population of Type II fibers (Teig, Dahl, and Tohrkelsen, 1978), whereas the PCA, in which Type I muscle fibers predominate, atrophies at a slower rate. These muscle difference in humans, however, may be smaller

than those observed in dogs.

Recurrent laryngeal nerve paralysis resulting in atrophy of the vocal folds is considered to be similar to that of Group 1 in this experiment. In this group of animals, the enzyme activities were partially decreased in the first month and the Type II muscle fibers were almost totally atrophied by the fourth month. Therefore, assuming that recurrent laryngeal nerve paralysis occurring in humans follows the same progress as in Group 1, it seems appropriate to institute treatment as early as possible to promote reinnervation and to prevent atrophy of muscle fibers. This position concurs with that posed by Sato and Yamada (1975), suggesting treatment be administered earlier to recurrent nerve paralysis showing atrophy.

Clinically, when an electromyographic discharge is observed in a case of recurrent nerve paralysis that shows no clinical atrophy in the vocal fold, the damage to the nerve is assumed to be slight, or it is believed that reinnervation has already occurred. This is similar to Groups 2 and 3 in this experiment. When the nerve is cut or crushed, the enzyme activity is less affected, so the metabolic function of the muscle fiber on the cell level exhibits little change. Therefore, in these cases, the prognosis is good. But even so, the recovery of function on the cell level does not always guarantee recovery of vocal fold movement.

In theory, the neuromuscular flap grafting technique (Sato and Ogura, 1978a; Sato and Ogura, 1978b) should offer the most promise for regaining vocal fold movement. In this procedure, the total nerve pathway is left intact, which is in contrast to the present experimental conditions where the nerve is damaged to varying degrees. Whether or not recovery following neuromuscular flap grafting is, in fact, greater than that after such nerve injuries as those in the present study is in need of further consideration.

SUMMARY

Histochemical changes in canine intrinsic laryngeal muscles occurring after recurrent nerve paralysis were investigated. The recurrent nerve was damaged surgically using three methods. The laryngeal muscles were histochemically examined every month following surgery for six months. Histochemical staining of serial sections was carried out to determine the presence of myofibrillar ATPase, phosphorylase, NADH, and SDH.

Results showed that following partial resection of the recurrent nerve, the activity of phosphorylase decreased rapidly and almost disappeared within one month after the operation. Activities of NADH and SDH dropped gradually but had not disappeared within six months of the operation. ATPase activity remained almost constant throughout the period of observation. When the nerve was crushed, enzyme activity did not change significantly. The degree of change in enzyme activity following section of the nerve was less than that after partial removal of the nerve. Fiber type grouping was observed predominantly following nerve section. This finding may explain the misdirected reinnervation of the laryngeal muscles that occurs in patients with recurrent nerve paralysis.

REFERENCES

Bajusz, E. (1964). "Red" skeletal muscle fiber: Relative independence of neural control. *Science, 145*, 938–939.

Barka, T., and Anderson, P.J. (1963). *Theory, practice, and bibliography*. New York: Hoeber.

Broeckaert, J. (1904). Uber der besondere Vulnerabilität des M. cricoaryt. Post. *Internat Centralblatt Laryng Rhinol Wissenschaft, 20*, 556.

Brook, M.H., and Keiser, K.K. (1970). Muscle fiber types: How many and what kind? *Arch Neurol, 23*, 369–379.

Davies, R.E., Goldspind, G., and Larson, R.E. (1969). ATP utilization by fast and slow muscles during the development and maintenance of isometric tension. *J Physiol, 206*, 28–29.

Engel, W.K. (1969). The essentiality of histo- and cytochemical studies of skeletal muscle in the investigation of neuromuscular disease. *Neurology, 12,* 777–794.

Engel, W.K., Brooke, M.H., and Nelson, P.G. (1966). Histochemical studies of denervation of tenotomized cat muscle: Illustrating difficulties in relating experimental animal conditions to human neuromuscular disease. *Ann N.Y. Acad Sci, 138,* 160–185.

Edstrom, L., Linquist, C., and Mårtensson, A. (1974). Correlation between functional and histochemical properties of the intrinsic laryngeal muscles in the cat. In B. Wyke (Ed.), *Ventilatory and phonatory control systems* (pp. 392–407). London: Oxford University Press.

Grabower (1909). Uber die Veranderungen in gelahmten Kehlkopfmuskeln. Ein klinischel Beiplag. *Arch Laryng, 21,* 340–356.

Gunn, H.M. (1972). Histochemical observations on laryngeal skeletal muscle fibers in "normal" horses. *Equine Veterinary Journal, 4,* 144–148.

Gunn, H.M. (1973). Further observations on laryngeal skeletal muscle in the horse. *Equine Veterinary Journal, 5,* 77–80.

Hall-Craggs, E.C.B. (1968). The contraction times and enzyme activity of two rabbit laryngeal muscles. *J Anat, 102,* 241–255.

Hirose, H., Ushijima, T., Kobayashi, T., and Sawashima, M. (1969). An experimental study of the contraction properties of the laryngeal muscles in the cat. *Ann Otol, 78,* 297–306.

Hogenhuis, L.A.G., and Engel, W.K. (1965). Histochemistry and cytochemistry of experimentally denervated guinea pig muscle. I. Histochemistry. *Acta Anat, 60,* 39–65.

Izuka, T. (1966). Experimental studies on the nerve interception and atrophy of the intrinsic muscle of the larynx. *Jap Jour Otol Tokyo, 69,* 176–195.

Karpati, G., and Engel, W.K. (1968). Corrective histochemical study of skeletal muscle after suprasegmental denervation. Peripheral nerve dissection and skeletal fixation. *Neurology, 18,* 681–692.

Lee, D. H. (1965). Studies on the nerve innervation of the larynx. Part II. The influence of nerve interception to the vocal cord muscle. *Jap Jour Otol Tokyo, 68,* 1208–1223.

Malmgren, L.T. (1981). Histochemical characteristics of muscle fiber types in the posterior cricoarytenoid muscle. *Ann Otol, 90,* 423–429.

Mårtensson, A., and Skoglund, C. R. (1964). Contraction properties of intrinsic laryngeal muscles. *Acta Physiol, 60,* 318–336.

Mascarello, F., and Veggettia, A. (1979). A comparative histochemical study of intrinsic laryngeal muscles of ungulates and carnivores. *Basic Applied Histochemistry, 23,* 103–126.

Murakami, Y., and Kirchner, J.A. (1971a). Respiratory activities of the laryngeal muscle and vocal cord motion in the cat. *Laryngoscope, 82,* 454–467.

Murakami, Y., and Kirchner, J.A. (1971b). Electromyographical properties of laryngeal reflex closure. *Acta Otolaryngol, 71,* 416–425.

Nachalas, M.M., Isou, K.C., De Souza, E., Cheng, C.S., and Seligman, A.H. (1957). Cytochemical demonstration of succinic dehydrogenase by the use of a new p-nitrophenyl substitute ditetrazole. *J Histochem Cytochem, 5,* 420–436.

Nachimias, V.T., and Padykula, H.A. (1964). A histochemical study of normal and denervated red and white muscles of the rat. *J Histochem and Biochem Cytol, 4,* 47–53.

Nagashima, T. (1970). An experimental study of recurrent laryngeal paralysis. — Electromyographic versus morphological findings —. *Otologia Fukuoka, 16,* 124–149.

Padykula, H.A. and Hermann, E. (1955). The specificity of the histochemical method for adenosine triphosphatase. *J Histochem Cytochem, 3,* 170–195.

Romanul, F.C.A. (1965). Enzymatic changes in denervated muscle. *Arch Neurol, 13,* 263–282.

Rosenfield, D.B., Miller, R.H., Sessions, R.B., and Patten, B.M. (1982). Morphologic and histochemical characteristics of laryngeal muscle. *Arch Otolaryngol, 108*, 662–666.

Ryu, S. (1982). A histochemical study of intrinsic laryngeal muscle. *Otologia Fukuoka, 28*, 394–402.

Sadeh, M., Kronnenberg, J., and Gaton, E. (1981). Histochemistry of human laryngeal muscles. *Cellular and Molecular Biology, 27*, 643–648.

Sahgal, V., and Hast, M.H. (1974). Histochemistry of primate laryngeal muscles. *Acta Otolaryngol, 78*, 277–281.

Sato, F., and Ogura, J.H. (1978a). Reconstruction of laryngeal function for laryngeal nerve paralysis. *Laryngoscope, 88*, 689–697.

Sato, F., and Ogura, J.H. (1978b). Functional restoration for laryngeal nerve paralysis and experimental study. *Laryngoscope, 88*, 855–877.

Sato, I., and Yamada, M. (1982). The waiting period for the performance of medical shift of the vocal cord for recurrent nerve paralysis. *Pract Otol (Kyoto), 55*, 1513–1516.

Seddon, H. (1975). *Surgical disorders of the peripheral nerves.* (2nd ed.) Edinburgh: Churchill Livingston.

Shin, T. (1962). An electromyographical study of intrinsic laryngeal muscles. *Pract Otol (Kyoto), 55*, 472–492.

Smith, B. (1965). Change in the enzyme histochemistry of skeletal muscle during experimental denervation and reinnervation. *J Neurol Neurosurg Psychiat, 28*, 99–103.

Takenouchi, T., and Kuriaki, H. (1955). Histochemical detection of phosphorylase in animals. *J Histochem Cytochem, 3*, 153–160.

Teig, E., Dahl, H.A., and Tohrkelsen, H. (1978). Actomyosin ATPase activity of human laryngeal muscles. *Acta Otolaryngol, 85*, 272–281.

Warmolts, J.R. (1981). Electrodiagnosis in neuromuscular disorders. *Am Inter Med, 95*, 599–608.

Wuerker, R., and Bodley, H.P. (1973). Changes in muscle morphology and histochemistry produced by denervation 3,3´-lminodipropionitrile and epineurial vinbanstine. *Am J Anat, 136*, 221–234.

CHAPTER 11

Contraction Properties and Histochemical Study of Cross-innervated Intrinsic Laryngeal Muscles

Fumihiko SATO
and Yasuo HISA

In general, methods such as end-to-end anastomosis, free nerve graft, intramuscular nerve insertion, and contiguous muscle transfer are performed for peripheral motor nerve paralysis and its consequent motor disturbance. However, in most cases the damaged nerve cannot be used. Contiguous nerve transfer or implantation of a nerve-muscle unit to the paralyzed muscle is sometimes successful.

The skeletal muscles are classified physiologically as fast and slow, and histochemically as high-oxidative (dark) and low-oxidative (light) muscles. The soleus muscle is a representative slow, high-oxi-

dative muscle and has usually been used as a control in the study of the contraction properties of successfully cross-reinnervated muscle. Since Buller, Eccles, and Eccles (1960) and Close (1965) reported that contraction velocity of fast and slow muscles was reversed after cross-union of the nerve controlling each muscle, Dubuwitz (1967), Romanul and Meulen (1967), Fex (1969), and Robbins, Karpati, and Engel (1969) have obtained similar findings from physiological and histochemical observations. Buller and colleagues (1960) reported that this phenomenon is influenced by the regenerated nerve, presumably mediated by axonal substances reaching the muscle fiber through the neuromuscular junction.

Our reports prior to the clinical application of pedicle nerve muscle grafting (PNMG) were designed as a basic technique for reconstruction of the neuromuscular system (Sato, 1974; Sato and Ogura, 1978a; Sato and Ogura, 1978b; Sato, Takenouchi, and Ogura, 1978). Using PNMG, we examined contraction and histochemical properties at the recipient site after cross-innervation in the laryngeal muscles and in the soleus and gastrocnemius.

MATERIALS AND METHODS

Cross-innervation

Preliminary experiment: Four mature rabbits were used. Under induction and maintenance anesthesia with intramuscular ketamine hydrochloride, we resected a 5 cubic mm piece of the left gastrocnemius along with the gastrocnemius nerve to make a PNMG. The gastrocnemius muscle block was implanted ventrally in the left denervated soleus muscle by suturing with 3-0 nylon. The direction of the donor muscle fibers was lined up with that of the recipient fibers.

Laryngeal cross-innervation: Eight mature hybrid dogs, each weighing 9-13 kg, were used. For PNMG, the superior laryngeal nerve and the cricothyroid muscle (CT) were employed because the contraction properties and histochemical characteristics of the CT were clearly known. The

animals were divided into two groups, each group consisting of four dogs.

Group 1: PNMG was implanted in the thyroarytenoid muscle (TA). Group 2: PNMG was implanted in the posterior cricoarytenoid muscle (PCA). Details of PNMG were reported elsewhere (Sato et al., 1978).

The cross-innervation was performed on the left side, with the right serving as the control. After confirmation of reinnervation by electromyography ten to sixteen months after the surgery, physiological and histochemical properties were determined.

Preliminary Experiment Group (Rabbits)

Under anesthesia with ketamine hydrochloride, the reinnervated soleus muscle was exposed, and the tendon attached to the trunk site of the muscle was cut and connected to a displacement tension transducer (F-D Pick-Up, SB-1T, Nihon Koden Co.) with a preamplifier (RP-2 for distortion pressure meter, Nihon Koden, Co.) attached (Figure 11-1). A gastrocnemius nerve was cut off at about 5 cm from the soleus muscle. At 1.5 to 2.0 cm from the muscle, the nerve was maximally stimulated and electrically stimulated via a bipolar platinum electrode. After physiological observation, the muscle was removed 1 cm from the nerve. It was stained by Nachlas's method and observed for distribution of succinic dehydrogenase in the muscle fibers.

Laryngeal Cross-Innervation Group (Mature Dogs)

Before contraction properties were examined, glottic movement during stimulation of the external branch of the superior laryngeal nerve was observed microscopically and recorded on 16 mm movie film for both Groups 1 and 2. Stimulus consisted of 1 V for 0.1 ms, taking muscular fatigue into consideration. Current spread to the neighboring muscle was prevented by using a mineral oil bath.

After completion of the experiment, the TA in Group 1 and the PCA in Group 2 were both carefully exposed and connected to a displacement tension transducer to assess their properties. Also, each muscle was taken at 5 mm from the nerve entry for studying muscle fiber distribution as shown by succinic dehydrogenase staining.

Succinic Dehydrogenase Staining (Nachlas's Method)

Muscle samples from the rabbit experiment and from the laryngeal PNMG experiment in dogs were checked for fiber distribution by the following techniques:

1. Fresh muscle pieces were cut into 10 μm sections with a cryostat.
2. The thin sections were dipped in a mixture containing 5 cc of 0.2 M phosphate buffer solution (pH 7.6), 5 cc of 0.2 M sodium succinate, and 10 cc of 0.1 percent nitro blue tetrazolium solution for 30 min at 37°C, washed with distilled water, fixed with 10 percent formalin, then placed in glycerin-gelatin.

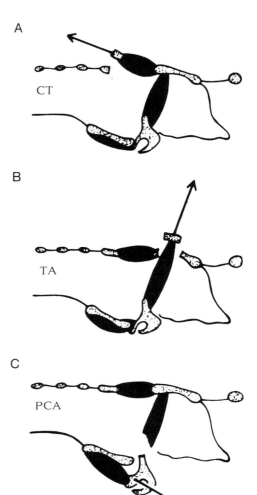

A

CT

B

TA

C

PCA

Figure 11-1. *Direction of force for tension transducer (F-D Pick-Up) connected to each intrinsic laryngeal muscle studied. A: CT, B: TA, C: PCA.*

RESULTS

Preliminary Experiment

In all four cases the graft took well and appropriate contraction was obtained with electrical stimulation of the gastrocnemius nerve. The contraction time ranged from 42 to 48 ms in cross-innervated soleus muscles, and from 57 to 79 ms in the control soleus muscles. These differences were statistically significant.

Generally, the soleus represents a muscle with high-oxydase activity. In the succinic dehydrogenase specimen of the rabbit (Figure 11-2), the muscle consisted of fiber groups of 15 to 30 μm in which foramazan precipitation was granular, and relatively equal throughout. The gastroncemius muscle consisted of 15 to 20 μm fiber groups strongly precipitated by formazan (called high oxidative or dark fiber) and 20 to 35 μm fibers with less precipitation by formazan (called low oxidative or light fiber). One year after the cross-innervation, the soleus muscle lost its original fiber distribution and its properties clearly changed into that of the gastrocnemius muscle, exhibiting a mixture of high oxidative dark and low oxidative light fibers as shown in Figure 11-2.

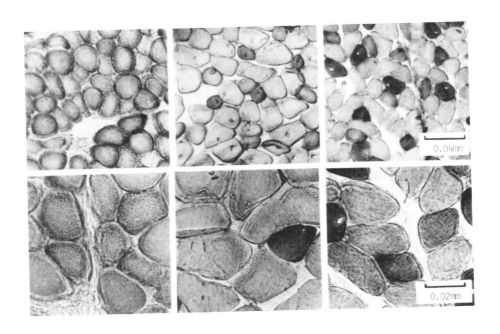

Figure 11-2. *Microscopic pictures of soleus, gastrocnemius, and cross-innervated soleus muscles (succinic dehydrogenase stain).*

Laryngeal Cross-Innervation

Contraction Properties

Table 11-1 shows the contraction properties of the three intrinsic laryngeal muscles in normal mature dogs (see Chapter 9). The CT was relatively similar to the PCA in contraction time. Table 11-2 shows the results of the present experiments. In Group 1, the contraction time of the cross-innervated TA averaged 36.3 ms and the fusion frequency 35 to 45 Hz. In Group 2, the contraction time of the cross-innervated PCA averaged 38.5 ms and the fusion frequency 35 to 40 Hz. The contraction properties of the cross-innervated muscles in both groups were, therefore, similar to those of the normal CT.

Glottic Movement Due to Electrical Stimulation of the Regenerated Nerve

Figure 11-3 shows the glottis during bilateral stimulation of the nerve innervating each normal intrinsic laryngeal muscle at different frequencies. The PCA showed maximum abduction at more than 40 Hz, whereas the TA showed the maximum adduction at more than 60 Hz. As the fusion frequency of

the two muscles was 45 Hz and 95 Hz, respectively, there was considerable energy available until the point where the muscle itself showed tetanic contraction. On the other hand, in the present experiment (Figure 11-4), the maximum contraction to adduction in Group 1 and that to abduction in Group 2 occurred at 30 to 40 Hz.

Distribution of the Muscle Fibers

The venter of the muscle was used for fiber size measurement. Distribution of the muscle fibers differed at the part nearest to the tendon and venter in this series. In the non-treated CT, TA, and PCA of the dogs, the fiber distribution after succinic dehydrogenase staining was not as clear as it was in the soleus and gastrocnemius muscle. However, it was possible to identify the quantitative properties of the fiber distribution of each muscle.

The CT exhibited a 10 to 25 μm fiber mass, and, unlike the gastrocnemius fibers, light and dark fiber types were indistinguishable by size. Even large fibers of about 25 μm, sometimes proved to be dark fibers with much granular formazan precipitation, whereas some small fibers of 10 μm were

Table 11-1.
Contraction Properties in Normal Canine Intrinsic Laryngeal Muscles.

	CT	TA	PCA
Contraction time	38 ms	14 ms	42 ms
Half-relaxation time	31.7 ms	16 ms	37.2 ms
Tetanus: twitch tension ratio	4.5	7.1	3.8
Fusion frequency	40 Hz	95 Hz	45 Hz

Table 11-2.
Contraction Properties in Canine Intrinsic Laryngeal Muscles After Cross-Innervation.

Tetanus twitch tension ratio	TA (in Group 1)	PCA (in Group 2)
Contraction time	36.3 ms	38.5 ms
Half-relaxation time	33.2 ms	30.9 ms
Tetanus twitch tension ratio	4.1	4.7
Fusion frequency	35 - 45 (Hz)	35 - 40 (Hz)

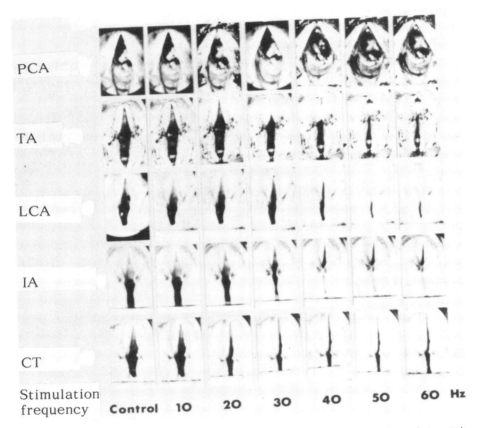

Figure 11-3. *Glottic views during bilateral stimulation of motor nerve branch to each intrinsic laryngeal muscle at different frequencies. PCA: Posterior cricoarytenoid, TA: thyroarytenoid, LCA: Lateral cricoarytenoid, IA: Interarytenoid, CT: cricothyroid.*

light. There were also fibers that showed an intermediate stain between the two.

The TA was almost totally composed of dark fibers containing intermediate fibers of 1 to 20 μm, with very few light fibers (Figure 11-5).

The PCA showed a fiber distribution that was morphologically similar to that of the CT. A mixture of fibers 10 to 25 μm was observed. Nevertheless, there were many more dark fibers in the PCA than in the CT (Figure 11-6).

After 10 to 16 months, the TA in Group 1 showed a distribution remarkably similar to that of the CT in that the number of light fibers in the 10 to 25 μm group had increased (Figure 11-5).

In Group 2, the treated PCA showed a distribution similar to that of the CT and the number of dark fibers decreased as compared with the non-treated PCA (Figure 11-6).

These results suggested that the physiological and histochemical properties of the re-innervated TA (Group 1) and PCA (Group 2) changed to those of the CT.

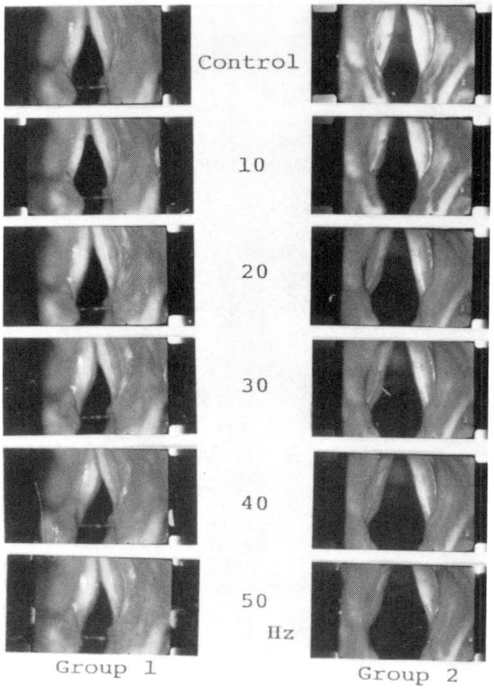

Figure 11-4. Glottic views during stimulation of nerve to cross-innervated muscles at different frequencies. Left side was operated upon.

DISCUSSION

There are two approaches used in investigating the properties of muscle undergoing cross-innervation: a physiological and a histochemical approach. Generally, a physiological investigation is made on the contraction properties of the muscle, whereas a histochemical approach is used to investigate the enzymatic activity and the distribution of the muscle fibers. In this paper, we investigat-

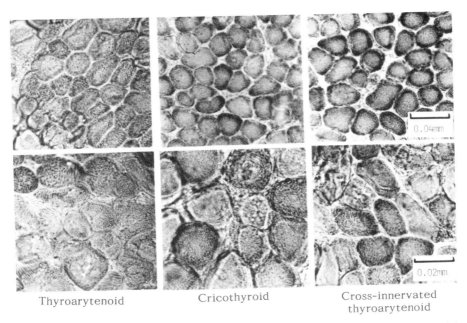

Thyroarytenoid   Cricothyroid   Cross-innervated
                                              thyroarytenoid

Figure 11-5. *Microscopic pictures of TA, CT, and cross-innervated TA (succinic dehydrogenase stain).*

ed the physiological and histochemical properties after cross-innervation by PNMG, a basic technique for reconstructing the neuromuscular system.

Since Buller and colleagues (1960) used the cat's soleus muscle in the study of cross-innervation by end-to-end anastomosis, rats, guinea pigs, and rabbits have been used (Buller et al., 1960; Close, 1965; Dubuwitz, 1967; Romanul and Meulen, 1967; Fex, 1969; Robbins et al., 1969). PNMG studies, however, have not been reported. Such cross-innervation studies should be done after complete reinnervation of the recipient muscle. This requires six months for end-to-end anastomosis, and three months for PNMG. Our studies were per-

formed ten months after the cross-innervation. The soleus muscle reinnervated by PNMG exhibited the properties of the donor, that is, the fast muscle showed a mixed type of high and low oxidative fibers. This was also true in many studies of cross-innervation employing end-to-end anastomosis. Therefore, the physiological and histochemical changes in the muscle undergoing PNMG could not be due to replacement by the donor muscle, but must be due to the influence of the reinnervating nerve.

Related studies concerning physiological properties of the intrinsic laryngeal muscles have been conducted in dogs (Mårtensson and Skoglund, 1964; Hast, 1967) and in cats (Mårtensson and

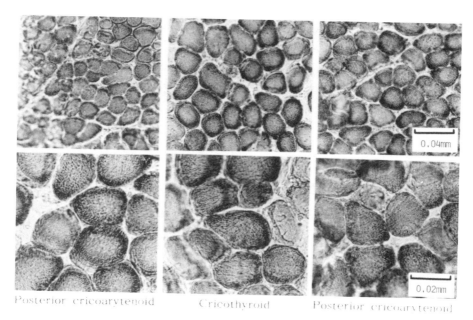

Figure 11-6. *Microscopic pictures of PCA, CT, and cross-innervated PCA (succinic dehydrogenase stain).*

Skoglund, 1964; Hast, 1967; Ushijima, 1968; Hirose, Ushijima, and Sawashima, 1969; Murakami, 1972). Glottic movement due to stimulation of a regenerated nerve has been studied by Takenouchi (1963), with particular attention to stimulation frequency. We determined the physiological properties of the muscle in normals and after cross-innervation. The reinnervated TA and PCA of the recipient site resembled the CT physiologically. Changes in glottic configuration ceased at 40 Hz, the fusion frequency of the CT. The properties of the intrinsic laryngeal muscle reinnervated by PNMG changed to the properties of the original donor muscle.

SUMMARY

A PNMG consisting of the superior laryngeal nerve and the CT was implanted into the TA or the PCA. The physiological and histochemical properties of the reinnervated muscle after PNMG changed to those of the donor muscle, being determined by the nerve innervating the donor muscle.

REFERENCES

Buller, A.J., Eccles, J.C., and Eccles, R.M. (1960). Interactions between motoneurons and muscles in respect of the characteristic speeds of their responses. *J Physiol, 150*, 417–439.

Close, R. (1965). Effects of cross-union of motor nerves to fast and slow skeletal muscles. *Nature, 206*, 831–832.

Dubuwitz, V. (1967). Cross-innervated mammalian skeletal muscle: Histochemical, physiological, and biochemical observations. *J Physiol (Lond.), 193*, 481–496.

Fex, S. (1969). "Tropic" influences of implanted fast nerve on innervated slow muscle. *Physiol bohemoslov, 18*, 205–208.

Hast M.H. (1967). The respiratory muscle of the larynx. *Ann Otol Rhinol Laryngol, 76*, 489–497.

Hirose, H., Ushijima, T., and Sawashima, M. (1969). An experimental study of the contraction properties of the laryngeal muscles in cat. *Ann Otol Rhinol Laryngol, 78*, 297–306.

Mårtensson, A., and Skoglund, C.R. (1964). Contraction properties of intrinsic laryngeal muscles. *Acta Physiol Scand, 60*, 318–336.

Murakami, Y. (1972). Biomechanics of muscle contraction in larynx. *J Otolaryngol Jpn, 75*, 800–808.

Robbins, N., Karpati, G., and Engel, W.K. (1969). Histochemical and contractile properties in the cross-innervated guinea pig soleus muscle. *Arch Neurol (Chicago), 20*, 318–329.

Romanul, F.C.A., and Meulen, J.P. (1967). Slow and fast muscles after cross innervation: Enzymatic and physiological changes. *Arch Neurol, 17*, 387–402.

Sato, F. (1974). Experimental investigation of laryngeal transplantation, Part I: Autotransplantation of canine larynx. *Pract Otol (Kyoto), 67*, 997–1011.

Sato, F., and Ogura, J.H. (1978a). Reconstruction of laryngeal function for recurrent laryngeal nerve paralysis. *Laryngoscope, 88*, 689–697.

Sato, F., and Ogura, J.H. (1978b). Functional restoration for recurrent laryngeal nerve paralysis. An experimental study. *Laryngoscope, 88*, 855–877.

Sato F., Takenouchi, S., and Ogura, J.H. (1978). Pedicle nerve muscle grafting. *Jpn J Transplantation, 13*, 105–109.

Takenouchi, S. (1963). Vocal cord movement by stimulation of laryngeal nerve. *Pract Otol (Kyoto), 56*, 399–420.

Ushijima, T. (1968). An experimental study of the mechanical properties of the laryngeal muscle. *J Otolaryngol Jpn, 71*, 1494–1509.

CHAPTER 12

Muscle Spindles in Human Intrinsic Laryngeal Muscles

Hiroshi OKAMURA
and Yoichi KATTO

T he laryngeal reflexogenic systems for respiration, deglutition, and phonation may be regulated by myotactic, articular, and mucosal reflexes. The afferent impulses in a myotactic reflex are discharged from proprioceptive mechanoreceptors (muscle spindles, Golgi tendon organs, etc.) in striated muscles. However, only a few reports have appeared on the presence of muscle spindles in the intrinsic laryngeal muscles in humans, and those reports are not consistent, especially on the number and distribution of spindles in these muscles. Moreover, the fine structure of each spindle has not been explored . Obviously, more detailed information of muscle spindles is necessary for understanding the function of the muscles in various types of laryngeal activity.

In the present paper, the authors report the distribution and dimension of the spindles in human laryngeal muscles examined by histological serial sections, and also their fine structural features as revealed by transmission electron microscopy.

MATERIALS AND METHODS

The materials consisted of intrinsic laryngeal muscles taken from human adult male larynges which were surgically removed because of cancer. The muscles examined were the interarytenoid (IA), posterior cricoarytenoid (PCA), lateral cricoarytenoid (LCA), thyroarytenoid (TA), and cricothyroid (CT). These muscles could not be obtained from a single larynx because of the extension of cancer into various parts of the specimen. Therefore, three larynges were necessary for preparing all the specified muscles.

At first, the organs were fixed with Karnovsky's fixative (4 percent paraformaldehyde and 3 percent glutaraldehyde in 0.1M phosphate buffer at pH 7.3) for 90 min. Each muscle was then removed from the larynx and cut into a few segments. These segments were again fixed with 3 percent glutaraldehyde for 90 min. After dehydration with ethanol, the specimens were embedded in JB-4 plastic embedding medium and serially sectioned transversely, the section thickness being 1.5 μm. The first section in each of the 20 groups was stained with Lee's methylene-blue-basic solution, and observed by light microscopy.

Some of the specimens were prepared for tranmission electron microscopic observation. The muscle examined was the central region of the IA. It was transversely cut into several segments about 2 mm long and placed in 3 percent glutaraldehyde for 2 hours. The specimens were post-fixed in 20 percent buffered osmium tetroxide for 2 hours, block-stained with saturated uranyl acetate in 50 percent methanol for 2 hours, and embedded in epoxy resin. They were cut into thin sections with a Porter-Blum microtome, stained with uranyl acetate and lead citrate, and examined by electron microscopy.

RESULTS

Muscle spindles were found in all the intrinsic laryngeal muscles except the LCA. Figure 12-1 shows a typical example of the muscle spindle, observed, in this case, in the IA. It is enclosed by the fluid-filled capsule and is composed of a bundle of specialized thin striated muscle fibers (the intrafusal muscle fibers).

Distribution, Dimension, and Location

The numbers and dimensions of the muscle spindles observed in the laryngeal muscles, which are tabulated in Table 12-1, varied in different muscles. The largest spindle found in the PCA was 1,780 μm in length, containing six intrafusal muscle fibers. The average length of the muscle spindles observed in this study was 1,002 μm and the diameter 79 μm at the equatorial region.

The relative numbers of spindles determined by conversion to 1 g of the average wet weight of the muscles were 6.5 in the IA, 6.2 in the PCA, 3.2 in the CT and 1.3 in the TA. Therefore, the distribution of the muscle spindles in both the PCA and IA was relatively ample in comparison with that in the other laryngeal muscles.

The locations of the muscle spindles were the medial edge in the PCA, the central region in the IA and CT, and the central and insertion regions in the TA.

Intrafusal Muscle Fibers

The numbers of the intrafusal muscle fibers are tabulated in Table 12-2. The maximum number of the intrafusal muscle fibers was six in the spindle found in the PCA. However, 40 percent of the spindles (5/13) contained only one in-

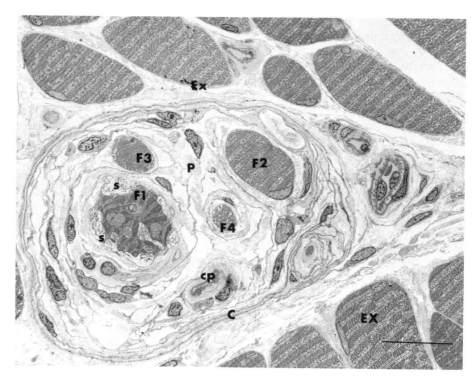

Figure 12-1. *An electron microscopic view of the muscle spindle in the IA. C: the capsule; F1 – F4: the intrafusal muscle fibers; S: the sensory nerve endings; CP: the capillary vessel; P: the periaxial space; EX: the extrafusal muscle fibers. The bar expresses 20 μm.*

trafusal muscle fiber. These fibers were classified into two types: nuclear bag fibers (NBFs) and nuclear chain fibers (NCFs). In this study, those two types of fibers were identified by the following criteria: When the diameter of an intrafusal muscle fiber was wider than 15 μm, or a fiber with a diameter of between 12 and 15 μm extended beyond the limit of the spindle capsule, it was considered to be a NBF, and the other fibers were judged to be NCFs. In the laryngeal muscles, the NCFs (Cooper, 1960) were more numer-

ous than the NBFs (Wyke, 1974). The composition of each fiber is also tabulated in Table 12-2.

Special Types of Muscle Spindle

In addition to the typical muscle spindle shown in Figure 12-1, the compound type of spindle and the monofibril spindle were also found in the laryngeal muscles. Functionally, a single encapsulated muscle spindle with the sensory and motor innervations is termed a single spindle or spindle unit.

TABLE 12-1.
Number and Distribution of Muscle Spindles in Laryngeal Muscles

Muscle Spindle	IA Diameter	IA Length	PCA Diameter	PCA Length	TA Diameter	TA Length	CT Diameter	CT Length
1	50	—	64	1060	40	870	40	440
2	45	300	85	1780	50	980	60	200
3	90	—	53	1300			40	1300
4	75	—	112	1590				

IA: the interarytenoid; PCA: the posterior cricoarytenoid; TA: the thyroarytenoid; CT: the cricothyroid. The values are expressed in μm.

The compound type of spindle is formed by two or more spindle units in parallel. Figure 12-2 shows the compound type of spindle found in the PCA, which consisted of two spindle units. One had two intrafusal muscle fibers and the other, four. At the polar region, fusions of the capsules and of the intrafusal muscle fibers were observed.

The monofibril spindle (Figure 12-3) has only one intrafusal muscle fiber within the capsule, and this type of spindle was observed in the IA, TA, PCA, and CT.

Fine Structure of a Muscle Spindle

By transmission electron microscopy, the fine structure of muscle spindles obtained from the IA was investigated (Figure 12-1).

The capsule of the spindle consisted of several layers of thin flat cells arranged in concentric lamellae, and was invested by a basal lamina. The thickness of the capsule ranged from 4 to 7 μm. This spindle had four intrafusal muscle fibers surrounded by the axial sheath without a basal lamina.

Two types of intrafusal muscle fibers were observed: the NBF, which contains an accumulation of nuclei in the equatorial region, and the NCF, which contains nuclei arranged in a row. F1 in Figure 12-1 was considered to be the nuclear NBF, as the diameter was large (21 μm) and several nuclei were observed at the equatorial region. F3 and F4 were thought to be the NCFs, as their diameters were small (shorter than 10 μm). Although F2 had a large diameter, an accumulation of nuclei was not observed. Therefore, it could not be concluded that this fiber was the NBF. In other words, the characteristic features of extrafusal muscular fibers were observed in this fiber.

The sensory nerve ending on the NBF was not a typical annulospiral ending, which is observed in a mammalian spindle. In three-dimensional reconstructions of the serial sections, it was an irregular coil ending with varicose swellings and branches of the axon. The axon terminals were not covered by Schwann cells, but enclosed together with the intrafusal muscle fiber by the common basement membrane. Most of the sensory

TABLE 12-2.
Number of Intrafusal Muscle Fibers

Muscle	Spindle No.	IF	NBF	NCF
IA	1	3	0	3
	2	1	1	0
	3	3	0	3
	4	2	2	0
PCA	1	3	0	3
	2	6	2	4
	3	1	1	0
	4	5	2	3
TA	1	1	1	0
	2	4	2	2
CT	1	1	1	0
	2	3	1	2
	3	1	0	1

IF: intrafusal muscle fiber; NBF: nuclear bag fiber; NCF: nuclear chain fiber; IA: interarytenoid; PCA: posterior cricoarytenoid; TA: thyroarytenoid; CT: cricothyroid.

endings were embedded in deep gutters on the surface of the fiber, some entering the sarcoplasm to terminate within the fiber.

The muscle spindle in the IA was also characterized by abundant collagenous fibrils which invested the intrafusal muscle fibers.

DISCUSSION

Wyke (1967) postulated that the servomechanisms of the larynx were carried out by three reflexes: myotactic, articular, and mucosal. Generally, the afferent impulses of myotactic reflexogenic systems originate in several types of sensory receptors found in vertebrate muscles. The simplest type is a free nerve ending, which is distributed in fascia, intramuscular connective tissue, and tendons, and is considered to be a pressure-pain receptor (Uehara, Campbell, and Burstock, 1976). Other types of sensory endings are more differentiated. These sense organs are known as proprioceptive mechanoreceptors, a group that includes muscle spindles, Golgi tendon organs, and Pacinian corpuscles (Uehara et al., 1976).

However, there has been no agreement concerning the presence or absence of muscle spindles in the human larynx . Formerly, it was said that non-weight-bearing muscles were devoid of muscle spindles, and that the proprioceptive mechanisms of the laryngeal muscles, if they exist at all, would be different from those of other somatic muscles.

Recently, the presence of muscle spindles has been demonstrat-

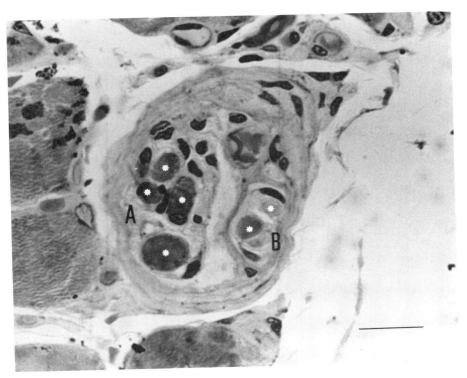

Figure 12-2. *A light microscopic view of the compound type of spindle in the PCA. One spindle unit (A) has four intrafusal muscle fibers and the other (B) two. The asterisks indicate the intrafusal muscle fibers and the bar, 20 μm.*

ed in the intrinsic laryngeal muscles in humans by several researchers (Goerttler, 1950; Paulsen, 1958a; Paulsen, 1958b; Bowden, Lucas Keene, Gooding, Mahran, and Withington, 1960; Koenig and von Leden, 1961; Lucas Keene, 1961; Rossi and Cortesina, 1965; Grim, 1967; Baken, 1971; Baken and Noback, 1971; Malannino, 1974; Wyke, 1974). However, their reports are not consistent, especially on the number and distribution of the spindles, and there are some reports that question the authen-

ticity of the reported spindles. For example, Zak and Lawson (1971) stated that striated muscle fibers within nerves might be mistaken for a muscle spindle. Moreover, the fine morphology of these structures in the muscles has not yet been reported.

Therefore, the authors investigated in detail the morphological features of spindles in the intrinsic laryngeal muscles in humans. As a result, they found spindles in all the intrinsic laryngeal muscles except the LCA. The spindles found in this study were typical encap-

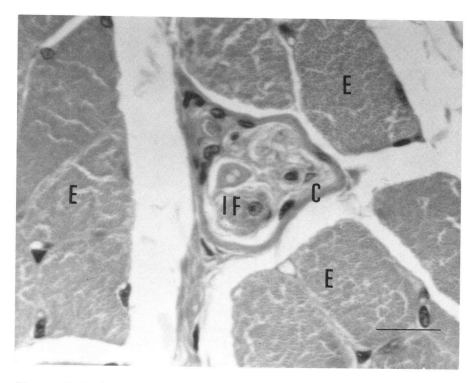

Figure 12-3. *A light microscopic view of the monofibril spindle in the IA. C: the capsule; IF: the intrafusal muscle fiber; E: the extrafusal muscle fibers. The bar expresses 20 μm.*

sulated receptors which contained a bundle of specialized thin striated muscle fibers, termed intrafusal muscle fibers.

Concerning the distribution of muscle spindles, a review of those studies in which they were evaluated quantitatively (Paulsen, 1958a; Paulsen, 1958b; Grim, 1967; Baken, 1971; Baken and Noback, 1971) revealed their presence in all intrinsic laryngeal muscles: in the TA (Paulsen, 1958a; Baken, 1971); in the LCA the IA (Baken,1971); in the PCA (Paulsen,1958b; Grim, 1967); and in the CT (Paulsen,1958b). Therefore, it is

reasonable to conclude that muscle spindles participate in a proprioceptive control of the laryngeal structures.

The average length of the muscle spindles observed in this study was 1,002 μm, and the diameter was 79 μm at the equatorial region, and the number of the intrafusal muscle fibers ranged from one to six. In comparison, their length in other skeletal muscles of the limb and trunk ranges from 3 to 12 mm and the maximum diameter is 250 μm. The number of the intrafusal muscle fibers ranges from 8 to 12 (Cooper and Daniel,

1956; Kennedy, 1970). Therefore, the dimensions of the spindles in the laryngeal muscles were relatively small in comparison with those in body muscles. These relatively small dimensions were comparable to those in the extrinsic eye muscles (Cooper and Daniel, 1949) and the anterior digastric muscle (Leenartson, 1979) innervated by cranial nerves.

As the index of the frequency of spindles in muscles, Voss (1937) proposed the relative number of spindles per gram of wet weight of the muscle. With respect to this index, Cooper (1960) divided the muscles into three groups: muscles rich in spindles, namely, 15 or more spindles; muscles with a medium supply of spindles, namely, from 8 to 14; and muscles with less than 8 spindles. From the results of the present study, the PCA and IA may be classified as borderline between those muscles with an average number of spindles and those with a small number of spindles. Therefore, the incidence of spindles in these two muscles is not particularly low. On the other hand, the TA and CT were poor in spindles. Grim (1967) reported that the relative number was 8.4 to 8.6 for the PCA. These results suggest that the muscle spindles in the PCA and IA might contribute in a certain degree to laryngeal self-adjustments. In other words, these two muscles may be categorized as slow and tonic, as a muscle spindle is a stretch-sensitive mechanoreceptor.

These assumptions are supported by the following two studies: (1) Using electron microscopy, Kawano (1968) found that these two muscles were rich in mito-chondria, a feature characteristic of slow, tonic muscles. (2) An electromyographic study by Hirose (1974) showed that the reciprocal function of the PCA during speech was performed mainly by the IA.

As special types of spindles, the authors found monofibril and compound spindles in the laryngeal muscles. According to Grim's report (1967), 20 percent of the spindles in the PCA were of the monofibril type. The present investigation also showed that 40 percent of the muscle spindles were of the monofibril type. Although this type of spindle is often observed in snakes and lizards, Cooper and Daniel (1949; 1963) found it in the extrinsic eye muscles and in the muscles of the limb and trunk at the site of transition of muscle into tendon. The compound type of spindle is numerous in the lumbricals and the deep cervical muscles (Cooper and Daniel, 1963). However, the function of these two types of spindle in the mammal has not been clarified.

The fine structure of the spindles in the laryngeal muscles has not been previously reported. The present investigation, using transmission electron microscopy, found that the capsule of a spindle in the laryngeal muscles was relatively thin in comparison with that of spindles in other muscles (Gruner, 1961). Generally, afferent impulses from the muscle spindle are triggered by passive stretch of the intrafusal muscle fibers, this, in turn, being induced by stretch of the extrafusal fibers. The fact that the capsule is thin suggests that compression of the intrafusal fibers by stretch applied to the extrafusal fibers is an additional afferent stimulus.

The intrafusal muscle fibers in spindles that respond to the stretch of the extrafusal muscle fibers play the main role for the stretch-sensitive mechanoreceptors. Those fibers are divided into two types: NCFs and NBFs (Cooper and Daniel, 1956; Boyd, 1960). Morphological and physiological studies suggest that the NBFs are more like slow tonic fibers (Uehara et al., 1976). In this study, the authors classified the types of fiber depending on the diameter and the extension of the fibers, as did Grim (1967) and Kennedy (1970). As a result, the intrafusal muscle fibers in the laryngeal muscles are found to be composed mainly of NCFs. However, their physiological significance is still unknown. In this study, one of the intrafusal muscle fibers examined by transmission electron microscopy resembled the extrafusal fibers. It is possible that an extrafusal muscle fiber itself entered the capsule during development of the spindle, or that the sensory endings that innervate an intrafusal fiber degenerated during their development and, as a result, an intrafusal fiber altered its morphological features.

The form of the sensory nerve endings that innervates the intrafusal muscle fibers is said to vary considerably, depending on the animal species (Uehara et al., 1976). The sensory ending in a mammalian spindle is an annular or spiral coiling around the equatorial region of the intrafusal fibers, termed the annulospiral ending by Ruffini (1898). However, the sensory endings observed in the IA were irregular coils with vari-cose swellings and branches of the axon. A similar type of sensory ending was found in the extensor digitorum muscles in humans by Kennedy, Webster, and Yoon (1975). The typical varicose terminal arborization is observed in a frog muscle spindle (Dogiel, 1890). Uehara and Desaki (1981) stated that the varicose terminal might be more sensitive to the stretch of the intrafusal muscle fibers than the annulospiral ending. As observed by the authors, the sensory endings in the IA contacted the intrafusal muscle fiber widely and entered the sarcoplasm to terminate within the fiber in part. These findings suggest that the sensory endings react more easily to passive stretch of the intrafusal muscle fibers, resulting in easily elicited afferent discharges.

Moreover, the muscle spindles in the IA had abundant collagenous fibrils that invested the intrafusal muscle fibers. These collagenous fibrils may be involved in protecting muscle spindles against traumatic stimuli such as pressure, or in regulating the ionic environment (Uehara et al., 1976). However, further investigation is needed to determine whether the type of sensory endings and the abundant collagenous fibrils thus described are characteristic of the laryngeal muscles.

CONCLUSION

By means of histological serial cross-sections, muscle spindles were found in all the intrinsic laryngeal muscles in humans except the LCA. The dimensions of the spindles in the laryngeal muscles were relatively small in comparison with those in ordinary skeletal muscles. As special types, the compound spindle and the monofibril spindle were also found. The distribution of muscle spindles in the PCA and IA was more abundant than that in the other laryngeal muscles. The sensory endings on the intrafusal muscle fibers were irregular coils with varicose swellings and axonal branches. The muscle spindle in the IA was characterized by its abundant collagenous fibrils that invested the intrafusal muscle fibers.

ACKNOWLEDGMENT

We would like to thank Prof. Yasuo Uehara, M.D. (Department of Anatomy, Ehime University) for his helpful suggestions and comments on this study.

REFERENCES

Baken, R.J. (1971). Neuromuscular spindles in the intrinsic muscles of a human larynx. *Folia Phoniatr (Basel), 23,* 204–210.

Baken, R. J., and Noback, C.R. (1971). Neuromuscular spindles in intrinsic muscles of a human larynx. *J Speech Hear Disord, 14,* 513–518.

Bowden, R.E.M., Lucas-Keene, M. F., Gooding, M. et al. (1960). The afferent innervation of facial and laryngeal muscles. *Anat Rec, 136,* 168.

Boyd, I.A. (1960). The diameter and distribution of the nuclear bag and nuclear chain muscle fibers in the muscle spindles of the cat. *J Physiol (Lond), 153,* 23–24.

Cooper, S. (1960). Muscle spindles and other muscle receptors. In G.H. Bourne (Ed.), *The structure and function of muscle* (pp. 381–420). New York: Academic Press.

Cooper, S., and Daniel, P.M. (1949). Muscle spindle in human extrinsic eye muscles. *Brain, 72,* 1–24.

Cooper, S., and Daniel, P.M. (1956). Human muscle spindle. *J Physiol (Lond), 133,* 1–3.

Cooper, S., and Daniel, P.M. (1963). Muscle spindle in man; their morphology in the lumbricals and the deep muscles of the neck. *Brain, 86,* 563–586.

Dogiel, A.S. (1890). Methylenblautinktion der motorishen Nervenendingungen in dem Muskeln der Amphibien und Reptilien. *Arch Mikr Anat, 35,* 305–320.

Goerttler, K. (1950). Die Anordnung, Histologie und Histogenese der quergestreiften Muskulatur im menschlichen Stimmband. *Zschr Anat, 115,* 352–401.

Grim, M. (1967). Muscle spindles in the posterior cricoarytenoid muscle of the human larynx. *Folia Phoniat (Praha), 15,* 124–131.

Gruner, J.E. (1961). La structure fine du fuseau du neuromusculaire humain. *Rev Neurol (Paris), 104,* 490–507.

Hirose, H. (1974). Functional specialization of the adductor laryngeal muscles with special reference to their function in speech. *J Otolaryngol Jpn, 77,* 46–57.

Kawano, A. (1968). Biochemical and electronmicroscopic investigation of the laryngeal muscles. *Otologia Fukuoka, 14,* 306–343.

Kennedy, W.R. (1970). Innervation of normal human muscle spindle. *Neurology, 20,* 463–475.

Kennedy, W.R., Webster, H.F., and Yoon, K.S. (1975). Human muscle spindles: Fine structure of the primary sensory ending. *J Neurocytol, 4,* 675–695.

Koenig, W.R., and von Leden, H. (1961). The peripheral nervous system of the human larynx. Part II; The thyroarytenoid (vocalis) muscle. *Arch Otolaryngol, 74,* 153–163.

Leenartson, B. (1979). Muscle spindles in the human anterior digastric muscle. *Acta Otolaryngol Scand, 37,* 329–333.

Lucas-Keene, M.F. (1961). Muscle spindles in human laryngeal muscles. *J Anat, 95,* 25–29.

Malannino, N. (1974). Laryngeal neuromuscular spindles and their possible function. *Folia Phoniatr (Basel), 26,* 291–292.

Paulsen, K. (1958a). Untersuchungen über das Vokommen und die Zahl von Muskelspindeln im M. vocalis des Menschen. *Szchr Zellforsch u Mikr Anat, 47,* 363–366.

Paulsen, K. (1958b). Ueber Vorkommen und Zahl von Muskelspindeln in inneren Kehlkopfmuskeln des Menschen (M. cricoarytenoideus dorsalis, M. cricothyroideus). *Zschr Zellforsch u Mikr Anat, 48,* 349–355.

Rossi, G., and Cortesina, G. (1965). Morphological study of the laryngeal muscles in man. *Acta Otolaryngol (Stockh), 59,* 575–592.

Ruffini, A. (1898). On the minute anatomy of the neuromuscular spindles of the cat, and on their physiological significance. *J Physiol (Lond), 23,* 190–208.

Uehara, Y., Campbell, G.R., and Burstock, G. (1976). *Muscle and its innervation: An atlas of fine structure.* London: Edward Arnold.

Uehara, Y., and Desaki, J. (1981). Comparative study of muscle spindle. *Adv Neurol Sci (Tokyo), 25,* 403–416.

Voss, H. (1937). Untersuchungen über Zahl, Anordnung und Lange der Muskelspindeln in der Lumbricalmuskeln des Menschen und einiger Tiere. *Z Mikrosk Anat Forsch, 42,* 509–524.

Wyke, B.D. (1967). Recent advances in the neurology of phonation; phonatory reflex mechanisms in the larynx. *Br J Disord Commun, 2,* 2–14.

Wyke, B.D. (1974). Laryngeal myotactic reflexes and phonation. *Folia Phoniatr (Basel), 26,* 249–264.

Zak, F.G., and Lawson, W. (1971). An anatomical curiosity; intra-neural striated muscle fibers in the human larynx. *J Laryngol Otol, 89,* 199–201.

PART 3

Neurophysiology

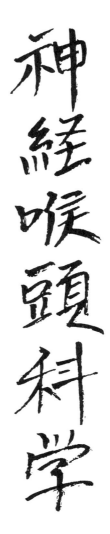

CHAPTER 13

Laryngeal Reflexes

Masafumi SUZUKI

The closure reflex is a well recognized basic function of the larynx. Various types of stimulation applied to the surface or deep structures of the larynx result in contraction of the intrinsic adductor muscles to prevent the entrance of a foreign body into the lower respiratory tract. Mechanical or chemical stimuli applied to the upper respiratory tract, innervated mainly by the fifth and ninth cranial nerves, also produce glottic closure.

In addition to this localized type of laryngeal reflex, various sensory stimuli originating in other parts of the body, both somatic and visceral, may result in reflex glottic closure if the stimulus is sufficiently strong or painful. Stimulation of the larynx may also result in changes in various organs, particularly those of the cardiovascular and respiratory systems.

It is very important to understand the mechanism of laryngeal reflexes that may be unexpected-ly encountered in daily clinical work. These reflexes include such things as laryngeal spasm resulting from direct stimulation of the larynx, respiratory disturbances resulting from large postnasal packs, and cardiovascular and respiratory disturbances such as bradycardia, decreased blood pressure, and respiratory depression resulting from laryngeal stimulation.

Another clinical factor known to have some effect on the laryngeal reflex is anesthesia. General anesthesia raises the reflex threshold but never abolishes it, whereas local or topical anesthesia act only on the receptor or afferent nerve function in the reflex arc.

The purpose of this review is to provide a neurophysiological description of the laryngeal reflex. The studies were completed during the last 20 years by Suzuki and Kirchner and their colleagues, using a variety of experimental animals, mainly dogs and cats.

These animals were anesthetized or paralyzed according to the purpose of the particular study. The details of each study will not be reiterated in this review. Readers interested in the specific methods and materials used are encouraged to review the original manuscripts; references for these are provided at the end of this chapter.

LARYNGEAL REFLEXES

Stimulation applied to the upper respiratory tract, particularly to the larynx, elicits strong reflex glottic closure. Its afferent input reaches the central nervous system (CNS) by the superior and inferior laryngeal nerves (Mårtensson, 1963; Kirchner and Suzuki, 1968; Suzuki and Kirchner, 1969a).

The internal branch of the superior laryngeal nerve (SLN) conducts most of the afferent impulses generated by receptors in the supraglottic portion of the larynx. These receptors are excited by touch or pressure or sometimes by irritant chemicals applied to the mucosa and by pressure or stretch stimulation to the deep tissues, including the cricoarytenoid and thyroepiglottic joint (Kirchner and Wyke, 1965).

The external branch of the SLN also conducts afferent impulses generated by touch or pressure stimuli applied to the anterior portion of the subglottic mucosa and the deeper structures, including the cricothyroid joint (Suzuki and Kirchner, 1968). Afferent impulses originating in most of the subglottic portion reach the CNS by way of the recurrent laryngeal nerve (RLN) (Suzuki and Kirchner, 1969a). All of these laryngeal receptors share the responsibility of eliciting the glottic closure reflex, the afferent impulse being transmitted to the CNS by one or more of these nerves.

The internal branch of the SLN contains many more afferent nerve fibers compared to the other two nerves, and when electrically stimulated, its threshold is lower than that of the other two nerves. The glottic closure reflex, in fact, is more easily elicited by stimulation of the supraglottic area than the subglottic.

The mechanism and characteristics of the laryngeal reflex can be examined in detail by electrophysiological techniques. When the central segment of the SLN is electrically stimulated, the reflex response is recorded from the adductor muscle or from its motor nerve. The latency of the reflex, when rectangular single shock of 0.1 ms duration is applied under these conditions, is between 7 ms and 20 ms in the cat and a little longer in the dog. When an electrical stimulus is applied to the central segment of the external branch of the SLN or RLN, a reflex response is elicited in the adductor muscle or its motor nerve fibers, but its threshold is two to three times higher and its latency is slightly longer than that of the internal branch of the SLN (Figure 13-1) (Suzuki and Kirchner, 1968; Suzuki and Kirchner, 1969a; Suzuki and Sasaki, 1976).

The laryngeal reflex is identifiable as a polysynaptic reflex by its long latency and by the partial or complete disappearance of the reflex response when a synaptic inhibitor (mephenesin) is administered.

In the cat, the reflex response can be recorded from the nerve to the contralateral adductor muscle, with 2 to 3 ms greater latency than that of the ipsilateral reflex. In the dog, a stronger stimulus is required (Sasaki and Suzuki, 1976). The greatest difference between the laryngeal reflex in the cat and dog is observed in the posterior cricoarytenoid muscle (PCA), which abducts the vocal fold. In the cat, when the central segment of the internal branch of the SLN is stimulated with suprathreshold single or repetitive stimuli strong enough to evoke reflex responses in the adductor muscle, reflexly evoked action potentials consistently appear in the PCA or its motor nerve fibers. It is possible that simultaneous reflex contraction of the PCA and the adductor muscle adds stability to the otherwise soft, fragile glottis.

By contrast, it is very difficult in the dog to record a reflex response from the PCA with the same level of stimulation that evokes the glottic closure reflex. Only a portion of the PCA contracts when low frequency (around 10 per second) and low intensity stimuli (subthreshold) are applied to the internal branch of the SLN. This reflex might be due to stretch receptors in the PCA or mechanoreceptors in the deep tissues. Similar action potentials can be recorded from the human PCA during high pitch phonation (Hirose, 1976; Sasaki and Suzuki, 1976).

Mechanical stimulation applied to the upper respiratory tract, innervated by the trigeminal and glossopharyngeal nerves, also

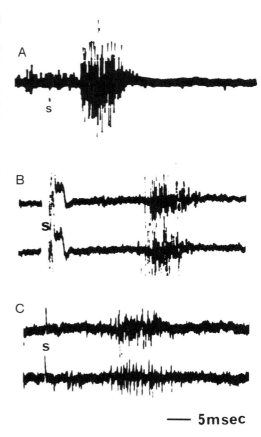

— **5msec**

Figure 13-1. *The reflex response evoked in the nerve to the adductor muscle by stimulation applied to the internal branch of the SLN (A), and the RLN (B), and the external branch of the SLN (C).*

elicits the glottic closure reflex (Murakami and Kirchner, 1972; Suzuki and Sasaki, 1977a). Afferent impulses originating in this area have almost the same effect on the laryngeal closure reflex as those arising in the supraglottic portion of the larynx. When an infraorbital nerve is stimulated electrically, the reflex responses recordable from the nerve to the adductor muscle show a low threshold similar to that in the internal branch of the SLN.

Postnasal packing, sometimes used to control bleeding after surgery such as adenoidectomy, may produce inspiratory dyspnea if the pack is too tight. This is caused by the continuous afferent input which elicits the glottic closure reflex which results in inspiratory dyspnea and delayed extubation. These problems can be corrected by changing the postnasal pack to one of proper size.

Many factors influence the laryngeal reflex. They include the type and variety of stimulation, changes of blood gas concentration, depth of anesthesia, etc.

A suprathreshold stimulus applied to the internal branch of the SLN elicits a consistent glottic closure reflex when it is applied less than once per second. When its strength is close to threshold, the reflex response is gradually diminished, possibly due to central inhibition. However, if there is additional sensory input such as subthreshold trigeminal nerve stimulation, the reflex response is recordable from the RLN and is similar to that resulting from a suprathreshold stimulus applied to the SLN. Thus, it may be a result of special summation in the CNS.

On the other hand, repetitive suprathreshold stimulation applied to the internal branch of the SLN elicits not only a reflex response in the RLN with each stimulus, but also elicits additional action potentials which are silent during single stimulations. This change in the laryngeal reflex might be thought to be the result of temporal summation in the CNS. When the internal branch of the SLN is electrically stimulated, the frequency that most effectively evokes continuous tonic contraction of the adductor muscle is around 10 per second.

LARYNGEAL SPASM

Reflex glottic closure is usually elicited by stimulation of the upper respiratory tract. Laryngeal spasm is also elicited by stimulation of the same area, but it should be distinguished from the simple glottic closure reflex.

Laryngeal spasm is clinically observed as a strong, prolonged closure of the glottis when the adductor muscle is tonically contracted. Tonic contraction of the adductor muscle can be experimentally produced by suprathreshold repetitive stimuli applied to the internal branch of the SLN. The electrical stimulus most effective in producing laryngeal spasm is that applied to the SLN at a frequency of 10 to 20 times per second. This results in an adductor motoneuron aggregate by means of temporal and spatial summation of sensory input. When the SLN, for example, is stimulated by a repetitive stimulus at a frequency of around 10 per second, the reflex response in the nerve to the adductor muscle is consistently synchronized with each stimulus. Additional action potentials are also recorded between each reflex response for a brief period (Figures 13-2, 13-3). Neither low frequency stimulation of less than two to three per second nor high frequency of more than 30 per second is effective. The reflex response evoked by high frequency stimulation is attenuated within a short period of time. Laryngeal spasm can be elicited by stimulation applied to nerves innervating the upper respiratory tract, and less easily elicited by stimulation applied to other somatic sensory nerves.

All of these changes in laryngeal spasm are modified in the CNS, where excitatory and inhibitory functions are variously controlled according to the character of the stimulus. The degree of laryngeal spasm is also changed with the lapse of time. The threshold for laryngeal spasm varies according to the respiratory status and level of anesthesia. Laryngeal spasm can be easily produced by lower threshold stimuli during hyperventilation and can be difficult to produce under deep anesthesia. Laryngeal spasm does not usually continue for long, because of progressive hypercapnia, which gradually raises the reflex threshold (Kirchner, 1970; Suzuki and Sasaki, 1977b).

It is of interest to note that laryngeal spasm is rarely observed in the newborn because of the immature condition of both the peripheral and central nervous systems (Sasaki, Suzuki, and Horiuchi, 1977).

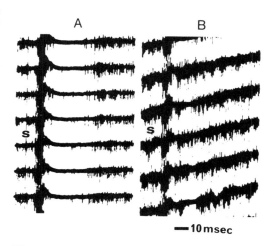

Figure 13-2. *Reflex responses recorded from the nerve to the thyroarytenoid muscle evoked by suprathreshold repetitive stimuli applied to the SLN at 1 Hz (A) and 8 Hz (B). Increased reflex responses and additional action potentials are seen in B.*

LARYNGEAL REFLEX AND RESPIRATION

One of the basic functions of the larynx is respiratory, by which both vocal folds abduct during inspiration to open the glottis. The nerve fibers to the abductor muscle (PCA) exhibit a rhythmic motor nerve discharge which is synchronous with the inspiratory phase of respiration. The vocal fold abducts just before contraction of the diaphragm. This can be demonstrated by simultaneously recording the nerve action potential to the PCA and phrenic nerve.

Respiratory rhythm is influenced by various types of stimulation applied to the upper respiratory tract. Complete apnea is elicited when the stimulation is sufficiently strong. The respiratory rate is decreased (or sometimes increased) when weak and continuous stimulation is applied to the upper respiratory tract.

Respiratory movement is centrally inhibited when the glottic closure reflex is elicited. A suprathreshold stimulus applied to the central segment of the SLN during the inspiratory phase inhibits inspiration for a certain period (several ms). This can be seen as the cessation of action potentials in the nerve to the PCA and phrenic nerve. Complete cessation of the respiratory movement can be observed when suprathreshold repetitive stimulation is applied to the SLN (Figures 13-4, 13-5). Although apnea continues as long as stimulation is applied to the SLN, the threshold for stimulation gradually rises, so that respiratory movement finally starts again,

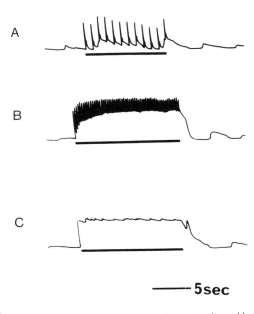

Figure 13-3. *Pressure recordings produced by vocal fold adduction elicited by repetitive stimuli to the SLN at 1 Hz (A), 4 Hz (B), and 16 Hz (C). A water-filled tambour placed within the laryngeal aperture was used.*

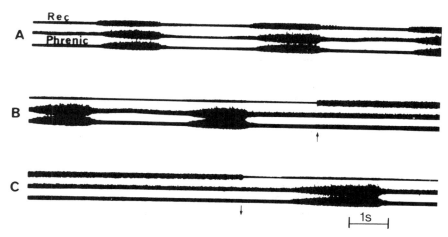

Figure 13-4. *Spontaneous action potentials recorded from the RLN and both phrenic nerves. A, B, and C are originally a continuous recording. A: Action potentials during spontaneous respiration. B: Suprathreshold electrical stimulation (30 Hz) was applied to the internal branch of the SLN beginning at the point shown by the arrow. A rhythmic discharge in the phrenic nerve is completely inhibited during stimulation. C: Action potentials in the phrenic nerve returned as soon as stimulation ended. Time scale 1 s.*

even though it is still weak and slow.

The threshold for evoking the glottic closure reflex is also influenced by various respiratory conditions. When an experimental animal is hyperventilated or well oxygenated, the glottic closure reflex is easily evoked by weaker stimuli. In other words, the threshold becomes low. On the other hand, if the animal is hypoventilated or hypercapnic the threshold becomes high, and stronger stimuli are needed to evoke the reflex (Suzuki and Kirchner, 1969b; Sasaki and Suzuki, 1976).

EFFECT OF VARIOUS SENSORY STIMULI ON THE LARYNGEAL REFLEX

Various types of sensory stimuli may influence the laryngeal reflex. Stimulation applied to the upper respiratory tract is, of course, the most effective in eliciting the glottic closure reflex, as compared to other sensory nerve stimulation. Nevertheless, somatic, visceral, or even special sensory stimuli can also elicit the glottic closure reflex.

Various sensory nerves have been stimulated to examine their effect upon the laryngeal reflex. When a central segment of a somatic sensory nerve such as the radial, intercostal, or sciatic is excited by a single stimulus, the adductor muscle of the intrinsic larynx contracts, and reflex responses can be recorded from the nerve innervating these muscles at a certain latency. Similar reflex responses can be recorded by stimulating a special sensory nerve such as the optic or chorda tympani. Acoustic stimuli (click sounds) also evoke the glottic closure reflex. This reflex is also elicit-

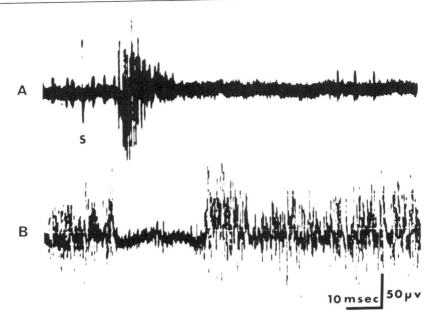

Figure 13-5. *Effect of the SLN stimulation on the laryngeal adductor and spontaneous inspiratory activity of the phrenic nerves. Reflex changes produced by a suprathreshold electrical stimulus (s) to the central end of the internal branch of the SLN. A reflex response appears in the adductor nerve in 10 ms (A) and the phrenic nerve activity is temporarily inhibited by the stimulus (B).*

ed by stimulation of visceral nerves such as the vagus in the chest, or the splanchnic nerve. The threshold of stimulation needed to evoke the reflex by stimulating these sensory nerves is generally higher than that of the SLN (Figure 13-6).

The different effect on glottic closure reflex produced by stimulating the SLN on the one hand and a somatic or visceral sensory nerve on the other is best demonstrated during repetitive stimulation. When the SLN is repetitively stimulated at just above the threshold, each stimulus evokes a consistent reflex response in the adductor nerve. The reflex response increases in duration and ampli-

tude and additional tonic action potentials soon join one response to another. The adductor muscle shows tonic contraction (laryngeal spasm) which becomes maximum at around 10 stimuli per second.

In contrast, when repetitive stimuli are applied to a somatic or special sensory nerve, the reflex response attenuates in a brief period according to increasing frequency of stimulation. When the vagus or splanchnic nerve is repetitively stimulated slightly over threshold, the reflex response attenuates in several seconds. The effect of the visceral nerve stimulation on the glottic closure reflex is relatively weaker than that of the SLN, but stronger than that of other somatic sensory nerve stimulation.

Although the closure reflex evoked by somatic or visceral sensory nerve stimulation is not particularly sensitive, and although some of it might be due to pain, it does, nevertheless, contribute to a widely varied reflex network which influences the protective closure mechanism of the larynx (Suzuki and Sasaki, 1977a; Suzuki and Sasaki, 1977b).

LARYNGEAL REFLEX AND CARDIOVASCULAR SYSTEM

Various changes in the cardiovascular system such as arrythmia, bradycardia, cardiac arrest, hematuria, and other disturbances of microcirculation may result from mechanical or chemical stimulation of the upper respiratory tract. In general, stimulation applied to the upper respiratory areas may produce moderate increases in blood pressure and pulse rate, but when excessively strong or irritative stimuli are perceived by the CNS, more serious changes in cardiovascular function may result. These effects are due to an increased outflow of autonomic, particularly vagal, nerve outflow.

When the central segment of the internal branch of the SLN is stimulated, reflex responses and increased efferent nerve activity can be recorded in the intrathoracic vagus nerve. Similar reflex changes can also be recorded during stimulation of an infraorbital nerve. This may be considered a laryngeal reflex in the wide sense, namely, a laryngo-visceral reflex (Figures 13-7, 13-8) (Suzuki,

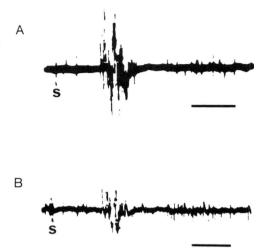

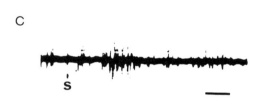

Figure 13-6. *Reflex responses recorded from the nerve to the thyroarytenoid muscle evoked by stimulation applied to the SLN (A), splanchnic (B), and radial nerve (C). Time scale 10 ms.*

1966; Suzuki and Kirchner, 1967;
Sasaki, Suzuki, Horiuchi, and
Kirchner, 1977).

Arrythmia, bradycardia, decreased blood pressure, and other
changes in cardiovascular function caused by a clinical procedure such as nasal or pharyngeal
surgery, direct laryngoscopy,
bronchoscopy, or intubation for
general anesthesia may be ex-
plained as a result of this reflex.
The effect of the reflex is usually
decreased under general anesthesia, but increased under light
anesthesia or during hypoxia or
hypercapnia. This reflex change in
cardiovascular function may be
the result of irritation (Reilly
phenomenon) or a vagal reflex.

POSTNATAL DEVELOPMENT
OF LARYNGEAL REFLEX

The laryngeal reflex mechanism
is not as mature at birth as other
neural functions of the body. Neural function develops over a long
period of time in humans, but develops in only a few months in the
dog. This makes the dog a good
animal model, because the reflexes of puppies of one day to two
months of age can be compared
to the reflexes of adult dogs. The
laryngeal reflex can be recorded
by a single shock stimulus applied
to the SLN even a day after birth,
but it is very weak, with a long
latency (about 35 ms), and with a
threshold about three times higher
than that of the adult. Nerve fibers
in the peripheral nerve are very
small in diameter, with very thin
myelin sheaths. For these reasons,
conduction velocity is very slow.
These fibers develop thickness

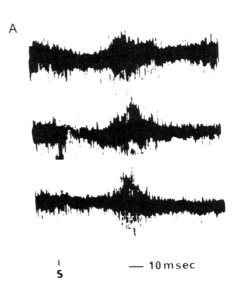

A

I
s   — 10 msec

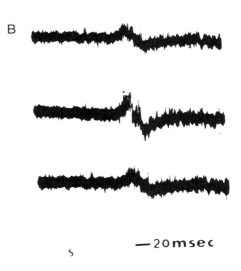

B

S   — 20 msec

Figure 13-7. *Reflex responses recorded from intrathoracic vagus (A) and splanchnic nerve (B) evoked electrical stimulation applied to the internal branch of the SLN.*

and myelinization day by day, month by month, so that they are almost completely developed by about three months after birth. The reflex network in the CNS is also regarded as functionally immature, particularly in its excitatory or inhibitory function. With continued neural maturation, the latency of the evoked response decreases despite increasing developmental length of the SLN and the RLN. This can only be interpreted as a consequence of progressive myelination and central synaptic maturation (Figure 13-9).

The major difference in the laryngeal reflex between the puppy and the adult dog is best seen during responses to repetitive stimulation of the SLN. During the first month of life, rapid attenuation of the primary evoked glottic closure reflex is produced during repetitive suprathreshold stimuli applied to the SLN. This observation is consistent with the difficulty of producing laryngeal spasm in the puppy.

This result suggests that laryngeal spasm does not occur easily in a newborn human. It might also explain why awake intubation or bronchoscopy can easily be performed in the neonate, and also why aspiration is often observed in the newborn. Mechanical stimulation produces only a group of single reflex adductions (Kirchner, 1970; Sasaki, Suzuki, and Horiuchi, 1977).

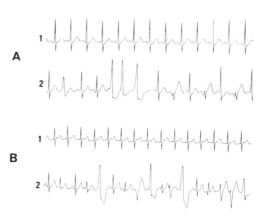

Figure 13-8. *ECG recordings from patients during general anesthesia. Multifocal ventricular premature contractions are observed just after intubation shown in 2. 1 shows ECG recorded before intubation. A: 37 year old female. B: 7 year old male.*

EFFECT OF ANESTHESIA ON LARYNGEAL REFLEX

The laryngeal reflex is variously influenced by anesthesia. Topical anesthesia inactivates receptors in the mucosa, local anesthesia blocks peripheral afferent nerves, and general anesthesia raises the reflex threshold in the CNS.

Under general anesthesia, the laryngeal reflex still remains active as long as spontaneous respiratory movement continues, but the reflex threshold rises according to deepening anesthesia. With single shock stimulation applied to the SLN, the reflex response is almost unchanged, but its duration and amplitude become shorter and lower than in the awake subject.

Laryngeal spasm is hard to produce by suprathreshold repetitive stimulation of the SLN under deeper anesthesia, but excitability of the laryngeal reflex is often increased under light anesthesia, or during induction or recovery from anesthesia. This might be the result of an imbalance between the excitatory and inhibitory functions within the CNS under these conditions.

This fact is important in daily clinical practice. Parasympathetic blocking agents, tranquilizers, and occasionally, topical anesthesia are useful in avoiding unexpected reflexes under these conditions.

CONCLUSION

The laryngeal reflex is a vital function of the larynx, and it is usually elicited by stimulation applied to the upper respiratory tract. However, reflex glottic adduction is elicited by other sensory input arising in somatic or visceral structures.

An extreme example of the laryngeal reflex is seen in laryngeal spasm, which is produced by prolonged reflex closure. Laryn-

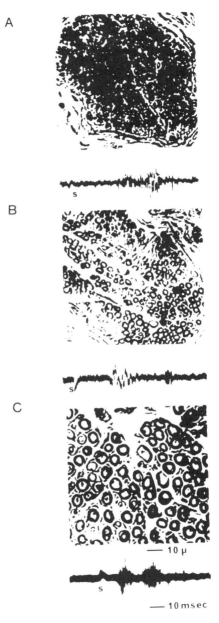

Figure 13-9. *Cross-sectioned display of RLN fiber size obtained at level of the second tracheal cartilage and adductor response to single-shock SLN stimulation. A: two days; B: 25 days; C: adulthood.*

geal spasm is observed when sufficient suprathreshold repetitive stimuli are applied to the upper respiratory tract.

Stimulation applied to the upper respiratory tract elicits not only reflex glottic closure, but also various effects on the respiratory and cardiovascular systems, such as inhibition of respiratory rhythm, arrhythmia, and bradycardia. Stimulation applied to the internal branch of the SLN which innervates the upper portion of the larynx is the most effective method of producing the reflex (Figure 13-10).

The laryngeal reflex depends on normal laryngeal function. When, for example, tracheostomy has been established for more than 2 to 3 months, the glottic closure reflex is suppressed, and aspiration of saliva or a foreign body may result (Sasaki, Suzuki, Horiuchi, and Kirchner, 1977).

The laryngeal reflex mechanism is poorly developed in the newborn, thus, laryngeal spasm is unusual because of immaturity of the reflex network within the central and peripheral nervous systems.

The degree of adduction during the laryngeal reflex closure varies according to the afferent input and to variations in the respiratory status and level of anesthesia.

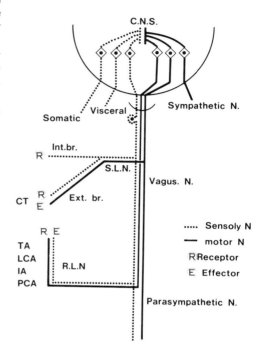

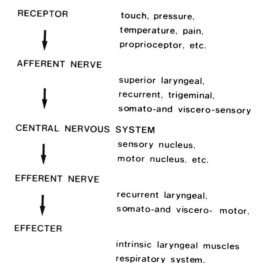

Figure 13-10. *Schema of the laryngeal reflex arc.*

REFERENCES

Hirose, H. (1976). Posterior cricoarytenoid as a speech muscle. *Ann Otol, 85*, 334–342.

Kirchner, J.A. (1970). *Revision of Pressman and Kelemen's Physiology of the Larynx.* (2nd ed.). Washington, DC: Amer Acad Otolaryngology–Head and Neck Surgery Foundation, Inc.

Kirchner, J. A., and Suzuki, M. (1968). Laryngeal reflex and voice production. *Ann NY Acad Sci, 155*, 98–109.

Kirchner, J.A., and Wyke, B. (1965). Articular reflex mechanisms in the larynx. *Ann Otol, 74*, 749–769.

Mårtensson, A. (1963). Reflex responses and recurrent discharges evoked by stimulation of laryngeal nerves. *Acta Physiol Scand 57*, 248–269.

Murakami, Y., and Kirchner, J.A. (1972). Mechanical and physiological properties of reflex laryngeal closure. *Ann Otol, 81*, 1–13.

Sasaki, C.T., and Suzuki, M. (1976). Laryngeal reflexs in cat, dog, and man. *Arch Otolaryngol, 102*, 400–402.

Sasaki, C.T., Suzuki, M., and Horiuchi, M. (1977). Postnatal development of laryngeal reflex in the dog. *Arch Otolaryngol, 103*, 138–143.

Sasaki, C.T., Suzuki, M., Horiuchi, M., and Kirchner, J.A. (1977). The effect of tracheostomy on the laryngeal closure reflex. *Laryngoscope, 87*, 1428–1433.

Suzuki, M. (1966). Influence of trigeminal stimulation upon the vagal outflow. *J Otolaryngol Jpn, 69*, 536–542.

Suzuki, M., and Kirchner, J.A. (1967). Laryngeal reflex pathways related to rate and rhythm of the heart. *Ann Otol, 76*, 774–780.

Suzuki, M., and Kirchner, J.A. (1968). Afferent nerve fibers in the external branch of the superior laryngeal nerve in the cat. *Ann Otol, 77*, 1059–1070.

Suzuki, M., and Kirchner, J.A. (1969a). Sensory fibers in the recurrent laryngeal nerve. *Ann Otol, 78*, 21–31.

Suzuki, M., and Kirchner, J.A. (1969b). The posterior cricoarytenoid as an inspiratory muscle. *Ann Otol, 78*, 849–864.

Suzuki, M., and Sasaki, C.T. (1976). Initiation of reflex glottic closure. *Ann Otol, 85*, 382–386.

Suzuki, M., and Sasaki, C.T. (1977a). Effect of various sensory stimuli on reflex laryngeal adduction. *Ann Otol, 86*, 30–36.

Suzuki, M., and Sasaki, C.T. (1977b). Laryngeal spasm: A neurophysiologic redefinition. *Ann Otol, 86*, 150–157.

CHAPTER 14

Laryngeal Proprioception

John A. KIRCHNER

Does the larynx possess a "position sense" similar to that which exists in the extremities, and which is capable of placing the vocal folds in a position which the singer knows, from past experience, will produce the desired sound once it is emitted? And at the moment the sound is emitted, is the necessary degree of coordination between the central nervous system, the respiratory muscles, the abdominal, pharyngeal, oral, and laryngeal musculature monitored entirely by the auditory apparatus?

The monotonous, unmodulated voice of the person who is completely deaf illustrates the importance of normal hearing in regulating vocal performance. On the other hand, the ability of a trained singer to produce a predetermined pitch at the moment it is emitted, often in the presence of high levels of background sound, suggests the operation of a receptor system in the larynx and other related organs which signals position, tension, and pressure within the various organs and structures involved in phonation. Such a system would be independent of any additional adjustments by the auditory apparatus.

The concept of a feedback system originating in the larynx itself is suggested by the following facts:

1. Mechanoreceptor end organs are present in the subglottic mucosa (Van Michel, 1963). Their thresholds indicate that they are capable of being stimulated by expiratory air pressures that develop during singing (Sampson and Eyzaguirre, 1964; Bartlett, Jeffery, Sant'Ambrogio, and Wise, 1976).

2. Muscle spindles and spiral nerve endings coiled around individual muscle fibers have been identified in small numbers in the larynx of animals (Abo-El-Enein and Wyke, 1966) and humans (Koenig and von Leden, 1961;

Lucas-Keene, 1961).

3. Large-diameter (10-15μm) afferent fibers in the recurrent laryngeal nerve constitute about 2 percent of its fiber population. This fact is compatible with the presence of a stretch-sensitive mechanoreceptor system in the laryngeal muscles (Gacek and Lyon, 1963).

4. Afferent nerve activity has been recorded from the superior and recurrent laryngeal nerves during excitation of laryngeal receptors by the type of stimuli that occur during phonation and singing. These stimuli include pressure (Figures 14-1, 14-2), vibration, passage of air across mucosal surfaces, changes in the length of the vocal cords, and stretching of the fibrous capsules of the cricoarytenoid and cricothyroid joints (Kirchner and Suzuki, 1968; Suzuki and Kirchner, 1968; Suzuki and Kirchner, 1969) (Figure 14-3).

5. These afferent responses are abolished by topical anesthesia applied to the laryngeal mucosa and to the joint capsules (Suzuki and Kirchner, 1969).

6. Electromyographic activity in the cricothyroid and thyroarytenoid muscles appears just before sound is produced (Buchthal and Faaborg-Andersen, 1964; Hirano, Vennard, and Ohala, 1970), suggesting a prephonatory "tuning" of the laryngeal muscles.

Although neural information undoubtedly arises within the larynx during phonation, and although it is carried centrally by afferent fibers of the superior and recurrent laryngeal nerves, the missing link in this chain of evidence is its effect on vocal performance. The problem is complicated by the existence of other feedback mechanisms in the intercostal and abdominal muscles (Bishop, 1973). Additional reflex mechan-

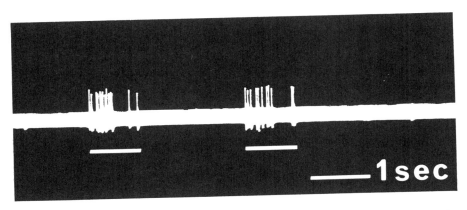

Figure 14-1. *Rapidly adapting afferent discharges recorded from a filament of the external branch of the superior laryngeal nerve during touch stimulus applied to the anterior subglottic mucosa (cat). Solid lines indicate duration of touch applied by tip of probe.*

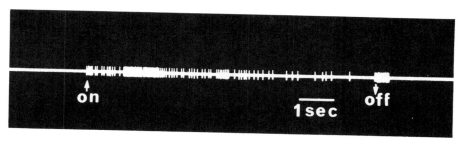

Figure 14-2. *Slowly adapting mechanoreceptor impulses recorded from a filament of the recurrent laryngeal nerve during light touch applied to the subglottic mucosa (cat).*

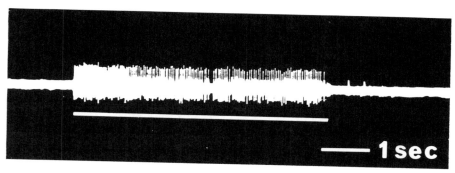

Figure 14-3. *Slowly adapting mechanoreceptor impulses recorded from a filament of the external branch of the superior laryngeal nerve during probe-tip stimulation of the capsule of the cricothyroid joint. Two percent tetracaine had been applied to the laryngeal mucosa to eliminate intralaryngeal stimuli (cat). These impulses were consistently abolished by 2 percent tetracaine injected into the joint capsule.*

isms exist in the muscles of the tongue, pharynx, and face, all of which probably contribute to a feedback control over the complex process of vocalization. A properly designed experiment would be difficult to perform in humans, the only animals capable of the type of controlled vocal performance that we define as "singing." And it would be equally or even more difficult in the experimental animal.

REFERENCES

Abo-El-Enein, M.A., and Wyke, B.D. (1966). Laryngeal myotatic reflexes. *Nature 209*, 682–686.

Bartlett, D., Jr., Jeffery, P., Sant'Ambrogio, G., Wise, J.C.M. (1976). Location of the stretch receptors in the trachea and bronchi of the dog. *J.Physiol 258*, 409–420.

Bishop, B. (1973). Abdominal muscle activity during respiration. In B.D. Wyke (Ed.), *Ventilatory and Phonatory Control Systems* (pp. 12–24). London: Oxford University Press.

Buchthal, F., and Faaborg-Andersen, K.L. (1964). Electromyography of laryngeal and respiratory muscles. *Ann Otol Rhinol Laryngol 73*, 118–123.

Gacek, R.R., and Lyon, M.L. (1963). The fiber components of the recurrent laryngeal nerve in the cat. *Ann Otol Rhinol Laryngol 85*, 460–471.

Hirano, M. Vennard, W., and Ohala, J. (1970). Regulation of register, pitch and intensity of voice: An electromyographic investigation of intrinsic laryngeal muscles. *Folia Phoniatrica 22*, 1–20.

Kirchner,J.A., and Suzuki, M. (1968). Laryngeal reflexes and voice production. *Ann N Y Acad Sci 155*, 98–109.

Koenig, W.F., and von Leden, H. (1961). The peripheral nervous system of the human larynx. II. The thyroarytenoid (vocalis) muscle. *Arch Otolaryngol 74*, 153–163.

Lucas-Keene, M.F. (1961). Muscle spindles in human laryngeal muscles. *J Anat 95*, 25–29.

Sampson, S., and Eyzaguirre, C. (1964). Some functional characteristics of mechanoreceptors in the larynx of the cat. *J. Neurophysiol 27*, 464–480.

Suzuki, M., and Kirchner, J.A. (1968). Afferent nerve fibers in the external branch of the superior laryngeal nerve in the cat. *Ann Otol Rhinol Laryngol 77*, 1059–1070.

Suzuki, M., and Kirchner, J.A. (1969). Sensory fibers in the recurrent laryngeal nerve. *Ann Otol Rhinol Laryngol 78*, 21–32.

Van Michel, C. (1963). Considerations morphologiques sur les appareils sensoriels de la muqueuse vocale humaine. *Acta Anat (Basel) 52*, 188–192.

CHAPTER 15

The Larynx-Lung Relationships

John A. KIRCHNER

The working relationship between the larynx and the lungs is well demonstrated in those animals in which primitive lungs first appear, like the lungfish and the frog. The frog, for example, having no diaphragm with which to suck air into the lung, must trap air in the floor of the mouth while the larynx remains closed, then "swallow" the air into the lung (Wind, 1970). And because the frog has no rib cage to provide rigidity, its simple sac-like lungs would collapse like deflated balloons during a deep dive, when external pressure is increased. But this collapse is prevented by the larynx, which, during expiration, closes partially or completely, thus acting like a cork in the neck of a soft plastic bottle. In this way, intrapulmonary pressure is maintained and the patency of intrapulmonary blood vessels preserved. The most primitive functions of the larynx, therefore, serve not only to exclude foreign matter from the airway, but to prevent collapse of the lung.

This mechanism has attained considerable refinement in higher animal species, including humans. Because of its ability to alter the area of the glottic aperture almost instantaneously, the larynx can act as a "brake" during expiration (Gautier, Remmers, and Bartlett, 1973). In certain types of dyspnea, the adductor muscles may contract voluntarily during expiration, and this may have some effect on the distribution of air within the lungs, or on the pulmonary circulation. This may explain the expiratory sigh and pursed lips of the emphysema victim. Similarly, the expiratory laryngeal grunt often heard in the newborn baby with respiratory distress syndrome may represent an attempt to maintain lung inflation and prevent collapse. In the eupneic state, however, active resistance at the glottic level is regulated entirely by variations in posterior cricoarytenoid muscle

(PCA) activity. During quiet respiration, adduction is caused by a gradual fall of tonic activity in the PCA and not by activation of the adductors (Figure 15-1) (Murakami and Kirchner, 1972).

The effects of pressure variations within the respiratory airway resulting from these moment-to-moment alterations in the glottic aperture have been well demonstrated experimentally. They exert an important influence on the depth and rate of respiration (Bartlett, Remmers, and Gautier, 1973) and are triggered by pressure receptors in the lung, in the subglottic trachea (Sant'Ambrogio, Mathew, Fisher, and Sant'Ambrogio, 1983), and possibly in the larynx itself. The larynx has two populations of pressure receptors, one of which responds to expansion, the other to collapse, both groups contributing to respiratory modulation. For example, negative pressure applied to the larynx increases the activity of the genioglossus and other muscles of the upper airway (Mathew, Abu-Osba, and Thach, 1982). Furthermore, topical anesthesia of the laryngeal

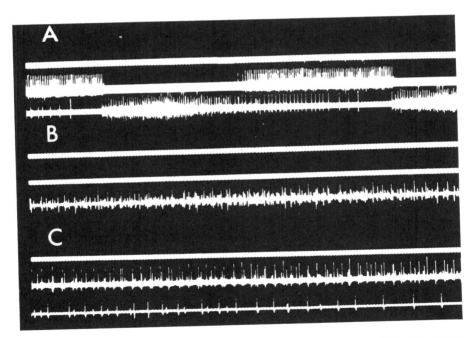

Figure 15-1. *(A) Quiet respiration, with slow time base. (B) Inspiration, with fast time base. (C) Expiration, with fast time base. In each of these three tracings, the top line shows EMG activity in the thyroarytenoid muscle, the middle line shows Expiration (EMG in the hypopharyngeus muscle), and the lower line shows EMG in the posterior cricoarytenoid muscle. The adductor muscle (top lines) is completely silent throughout the respiratory cycle, whereas the posterior cricoarytenoid (lower lines) contracts to some degree even during expiration, as shown in (C).*

mucosa or bilateral superior laryngeal nerve section abolishes the afferent nerve responses elicited by positive or negative pressures applied to the larynx, as shown by experiments reported by Mathew and associates (Mathew, Sant'Ambrogio, Fisher, and Sant'Ambrogio, 1984)

Although approximately one-sixth of the "pulmonary" receptors are located in the subglottic and upper tracheal mucosa, it is primarily those receptors located in the more peripheral parts of the lung that influence glottic aperture during respiration (Rattenborg, 1961; Bartlett, Jeffery, Sant'Ambrogio, and Wise, 1976; Remmers

and Bartlett, 1977), as inspiratory contractions of the PCA can be abolished by inflating the lung through a tracheotomy cannula. These influences are mediated by afferent fibers of the vagus nerves. After vagal de-afferentation, neither inflation nor deflation of the lung affect the level of spontaneous respiratory activity in the PCA (Figure 15-2) (Fukuda, Sasaki, and Kirchner, 1973; McCaffrey and Kern, 1980).

Tracheotomy, by reducing respiratory resistance, gradually abolishes the phasic inspiratory contraction of the PCA (Sasaki, Fukuda and Kirchner, 1973). This mechanism is probably responsi-

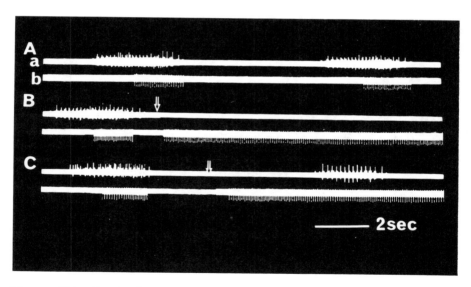

Figure 15-2. *Vagal afferent influences on inspiratory activity of the posterior cricoarytenoid muscle. In each of the three tracings, (a) = EMG in posterior cricoarytenoid muscle; (b) = Afferent discharges in left vagus nerve. (A) Quiet respiration. (B) At arrow, the lung was mechanically inflated. PCA activity stops at once, and vagal afferent potentials start, continuing as long as the lung remains inflated. (C) Same procedure as in (B), but after additional section of the right vagus beyond origin of recurrent laryngeal nerve. With complete vagal interruption, inflation of the lung (arrow) induces afferent vagal potentials, but the right PCA continues its phasic activity.*

ble for many instances of difficult decannulation after tracheotomy, particularly in the infant. It also explains why adding gradually increasing resistance to the airway by inserting partial corks into the cannula helps to reestablish laryngeal abductor activity and allow decannulation (Kirchner, 1982).

Tracheotomy-induced inactivation of the PCA can contribute to the development of subglottic stenosis. For example, when tracheotomy is performed after a period of endotracheal intubation, the increased risk of subglottic stenosis is due to (1) tube-induced abrasion of the mucosal surface at the glottic or subglottic level, in addition to (2) infection of this area by contamination carried upward from the tracheotomy site (Sasaki, Horiuchi, and Koss, 1979). Even the vocal folds themselves can become fused together through this mechanism if the abrasion occurs at the glottic, rather than the subglottic level (Kirchner and Sasaki, 1973).

A question that continues to puzzle the laryngologist is why the paralyzed vocal fold may occupy a partly abducted or intermediate position in a case of aortic aneurysm or cancer of the upper mediastinum. In such a case, the motor innervation of the cricothyroid muscle, arising from the vagus nerve high in the neck, is morphologically intact. This muscle ordinarily brings the vocal fold to the midline or near it, when the recurrent nerve alone is interrupted (Figure 15-3) (Suzuki, Kirchner, and Murakami, 1970). Electromyographic studies suggest that this type of glottal incompetence results from physiological inactivation of the cricothyroid muscle

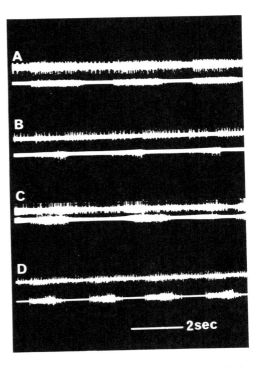

Figure 15-3. *Cricothyroid muscle activity in recurrent nerve paralysis. (A, B, C, D,): Four different cats, all having had section of both recurrent laryngeal nerves (light anesthesia). Upper trace in each: EMG activity in cricothyroid muscle. Lower trace in each: Inspiration (EMG of diaphragm).*

All animals were dyspneic, and the cricothyroid muscle in each case shows increased activity during both inspiration and expiration. These tracings show that the continuous activity of the cricothyroid muscle in bilateral midline vocal fold paralysis is the result of alternating activity of motor units which are active during inspiration and others which are active during expiration.

when both the vagus and recurrent nerves are interrupted. In this circumstance, vagal afferent information originating in pulmonary receptors is interrupted, and can no longer exert its monitoring influence over the cricothyroid activity (Figure 15-4) (Fukuda and Kirchner, 1972).

In the final analysis, however, the major influence over reflex laryngeal movements is the carbon dioxide content of the blood at any moment (Figure 15-5) (Fukuda and Kirchner, 1972). Widening of the glottis occurs during rhythmic bursts of activity in the recurrent laryngeal nerve. This rhythmicity, like that in the phrenic nerve, is accentuated by hypercapnia and ventilatory obstruction, and depressed by hyperventilation and resultant hypocapnia (Suzuki and Kirchner, 1969). Other respiratory reflexes, including those described previously, are of secondary importance, and serve a modulatory, rather than regulatory function.

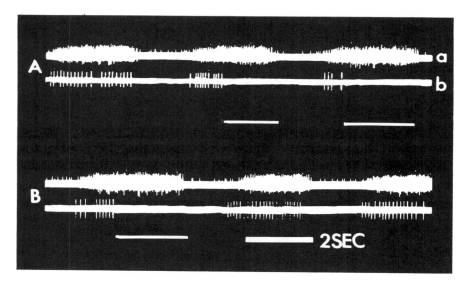

Figure 15-4. *Inhibition of cricothyroid muscle activity by blockade of afferent vagal stimuli. (A) and (B) are continuous recordings. (a) Inspiration (EMG of external intercostal muscle). (b) Cricothyroid EMG. Solid lines show duration of vagal blockade.*

Cricothyroid activity is inhibited only during interruption of vagal afferent impulses, accomplished in this case by tension applied to the vagus by a silk ligature. Similar inhibition of cricothyroid activity was observed when the vagus was blocked by 2 percent tetracaine or by being pinched with fine forceps.

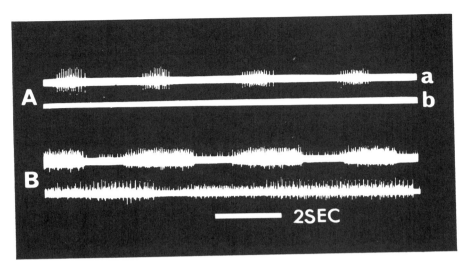

Figure 15-5. *Showing the overriding effect of hypercapnia. Moderate to deep anesthesia. (a) Inspiration (EMG of external intercostal muscle). (b) Cricothyroid EMG. (A) After tracheotomy is obstructed, there is no cricothyroid muscle activity at first. (B) After about 70 s of obstruction, irregular activity appears in the cricothyroid and persists in spite of pressure applied to the ipsilateral vagus nerve throughout the duration of this tracing. pCO2 at this time was over 40 mm Hg.*

REFERENCES

Bartlett D., Jr, Jeffery,P., Sant'Ambrogio,G., and Wise, J.C.M. (1976). Location of stretch receptors in the trachea and bronchi of the dog. *J Physiol: 258*, 409–420.

Bartlett, D. Jr., Remmers, J.E., and Gautier, H. (1973). Laryngeal regulation of respiratory airflow. *Respiration Physiology 18*, 194–204.

Fukuda, H., and Kirchner, J.A. (1972). Changes in the respiratory activity of the cricothyroid muscle with intrathoracic interruption of the vagus nerve. *Ann Otol Rhinol Laryngol 81*, 532–538.

Fukuda,H., Sasaki, C.T, and Kirchner, J.A. (1973). Vagal afferent influences on the phasic activity of the posterior cricoarytenoid muscle. *Acta Otolaryngol 75*, 112–118.

Gautier, H., Remmers, J.E. and Bartlett, D. (1973). Control of the duration of expiration. *Respiration Physiology 18*, 205–224.

Kirchner, J.A. (1982). Semon's Law a century later. *J Laryngol Otol 96*, 645–657.

Kirchner, J.A., and Sasaki, C.T. (1973). Fusion of the vocal cords following intubation and tracheostomy. *Tr Am Acad Ophth and Otol 77*, 88–91.

Mathew, O.P., Abu-Osba, Y.K., and Thach, B.T. (1982). Influence of upper airway pressure changes on genioglossus muscle respiratory activity. *J Appl Physiol 52*, 438–444.

Mathew, O.P., Sant'Ambrogio, G., Fisher, J.T., and Sant'Ambrogio, F.B. (1984). Laryngeal pressure receptors. *Respiration Physiology 57*, 113–122.

McCaffrey, T.V., and Kern, E.B. (1980). Laryngeal regulation of airway resistance. II. Pulmonary receptor reflexes. *Ann Otol Rhinol Laryngol 89*, 462–466.

Murakami, Y, and Kirchner, J.A. (1972). Respiratory movements of the vocal cords. *Laryngoscope 82*, 454–467.

Rattenborg, C. (1961). Laryngeal regulation of respiration. *Acta Anaesthesiol Scand 5*, 129–140.

Remmers, J.E., and Bartlett, D. (1977). Reflex control of expiratory airflow and duration. *Jour Applied Physiol, 42*, 80–87.

Sant'Ambrogio, G.,Mathew, O.P., Fisher, J.T., and Sant'Ambrogio, F.B. (1983). Laryngeal receptors responding to transmural pressure, airflow and local muscle activity. *Respiration Physiology 54*, 317–330.

Sasaki, C.T., Fukuda, H., and Kirchner, J.A. (1973). Laryngeal abductor activity in response to varying ventilatory resistance. *Tr Am Acad Ophth and Otol 77*, 403–410.

Sasaki, C.T., Horiuchi, M., and Koss, N. (1979). Tracheostomy-related subglottic stenosis: Bacteriologic pathogenesis. *Laryngoscope 89*, 857–865.

Suzuki, M., and Kirchner, J.A. (1969). The posterior cricoarytenoid as an inspiratory muscle. *Ann Otol Rhinol Laryngol 78*, 849–863.

Suzuki, M., Kirchner, J.A., and Murakami, Y. (1970). The cricothyroid as a respiratory muscle. *Ann Otol Rhinol Laryngol 79*, 976–984.

Wind, J. (1970). *On the phylogeny and the ontogeny of the human larynx.* Groningen: Wolters-Noordhoff Publishing.

CHAPTER 16

Brainstem Response Evoked by the Laryngeal Reflex

Yutaka ISOGAI,
Masafumi SUZUKI,
and Shigeji SAITO

T he laryngeal reflex is poly-synaptic through the central nervous system. Little is known, however, about the physiological mechanism and synaptic arc. The aim of this research is to study the synaptic circuit of the laryngeal reflex electrophysiologically, utilizing the averaging method with a far field recording technique. The principle of the averaging method is to improve the sound-to-noise (S/N) ratio by averaging, and to extract the masked input signal which is synchronized to the trigger pulse found within noise. By this principle, the signal component which is synchronized to the trigger pulse can be amplified and extracted from the noise component. The laryngeal reflex is known as a phase-lock reflex whose latency is several ms (Kirchner and Suzuki, 1968; Suzuki and Sasaki,

1976). Thus, if the firings of neural nuclei which are evoked by the laryngeal reflex are synchronized to the excitation of the internal superior laryngeal nerve, the brain stem response can be recorded. The brain stem response evoked by the laryngeal reflex will hereafter be called the laryngeal brain stem response (LBSR).

MATERIALS AND METHODS

Experiments were performed on adult cats, anesthetized with intra-peritoneal injection of ketamine (20 mg/kg/body weight). After trache-ostomy, the cats were immobilized by intravenous injection of pancronium bromide (0.25 mg/whole body weight). Artificial respiration (Narishige AR-1) was provided through a tracheal cannula during the experiment. The internal branch of the right superior laryngeal and the recurrent laryngeal nerve were exposed, and the sheaths of both nerves were dissected as much as possible under an operating microscope. Electrical stimulation (Nihon Koden, SEN7103, 0.1 ms duration) was delivered to the right superior laryngeal nerve through the isolator (Nihon Koden, SS302j) and the reflex potential on the right recurrent laryngeal nerve was monitored by a hooked bipolar platinum electrode. Simultaneously, the brain stem response was recorded by the averaging computer (Nihon Koden, ATAC350) connected to the differential pre-amplifiers (Nihon Koden, AB-671V, time const. 0.01″, high cut filter 1 kHz) through insulated stainless steel needle electrodes. These were inserted into the epipharynx (+) orally, cervical vertebra (-), and cervical muscles (g). The averager was triggered by a pulse of electrical stimuli to the superior laryngeal nerve. A block diagram of the experimental apparatus is shown in Figure 16-1.

Four groups of experiments were conducted:

1. LBSR was investigated under normal conditions. Effects of the stimulus voltage and the stimulus interval were studied.
2. Effects of respiratory conditions such as hyperventilation and hypoventilation on LBSR were investigated.
3. Origin of earlier components of LBSR was determined.
4. Effects on LBSR of removing the cerebellum were studied.

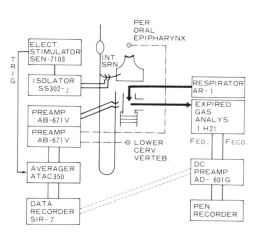

Figure 16-1. _Block diagram of the experiments._

In the latter three groups of experiments, ventilatory status was monitored by a gas analyzer (Sanei, I-H).

RESULTS

Experiment I: LBSR Evoked by the Laryngeal Reflex

LBSR obtained by changing the stimulus voltage while the stimulus interval was kept constant is shown in Figure 16-2. M. I. = stimulus interval. Figures in the left margin refer to stimulus voltage. Each tracing shows both of the responses, the right recurrent laryngeal nerve (upper trace) and the brain stem response (lower trace).

LBSR was recorded as four positive waves termed P_1-P_4, and four negative waves termed N_1-N_4. At any stimulus interval, the amplitude and latency of response were essentially unchanged at different voltages.

LBSR obtained during changes in stimulus interval, but at constant voltage, is shown in Figure 16-3. Changing the stimulus interval resulted in response patterns similar to those obtained by changing the voltage. With subthreshold stimulation, the amplitude of N_4 was rather obscure. This was related to the small responses of the recurrent laryngeal nerve.

P_1 latency was 0.5–1 ms, P_2 latency 1.6–2.3 ms, P_3 latency 2.8–3.2 ms, and P_4 latency varied according to stimulus conditions. N_1 latency was 1.2–1.4 ms, N_2 latency 2.4–2.7 ms, N_3 latency 3.4–3.6 ms, N_4 latency 5–5.5 ms.

Experiment II: Effect of Respiratory Condition on LBSR

In this experiment, respiratory conditions were changed by adjusting the ventilatory volume and frequency. Expired gas (FeO_2, $FeCO_2$) was monitored by an expired gas analyzer (Sanei, 1-H). LBSR showed no changes in the condition of hyperventilation, but did show changes in the condition of hypoventilation. The results are shown in Figures 16-4, 16-5, and 16-6.

In Figure 16-4, the upper traces in the left column show the action potentials of the recurrent laryngeal nerve. The lower trace is the LBSR. Numbers refer to the sequential time course.

In the first few traces, laryngeal reflex is kept constant, and LBSR is recorded normally. At No.5, N_4 becomes broad and obscure. At No.10, the laryngeal reflex disappears. At No.11, the P_4 component disappears. At No.17, the P_3 component becomes smaller. At No.18, P_3 has disappeared. At No.19, P_2 has also disappeared. In this figure, hypoventilation causes a decline in LBSR in the later responses.

Latency distribution data from Figure 16-4 are shown in Figure 16-5. As the latency elongates, the response disappears from later components.

In another case (Figure 16-6), at tracing No.10, the laryngeal reflex disappears, and LBSR is recorded only between P_1 and P_3. From No.11, the P_2 component also becomes flat. From this point, the amplitude of N_1–P_1 becomes smaller gradually. Simultaneously, the elongation of N_1 latency oc-

A

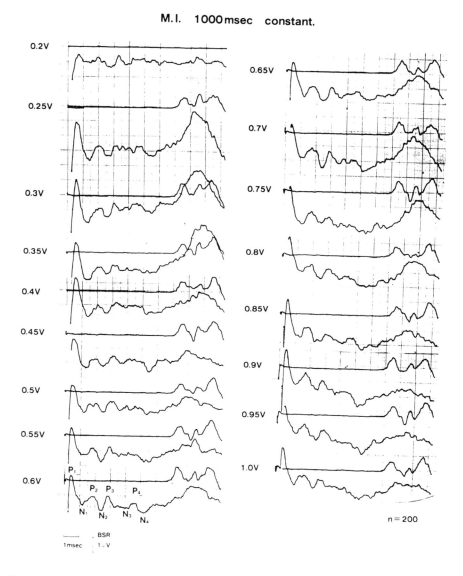

Figure 16-2. *LBSR obtained by changing the stimulus voltage while the stimulus interval was kept constant. M.I. = stimulus interval. Figures in the left margin refer to stimulus*

B

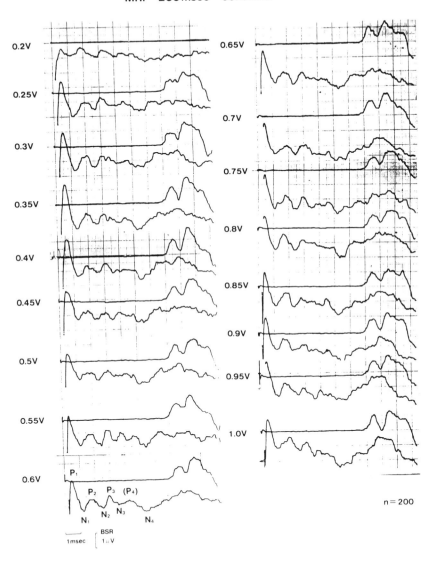

voltage. Each tracing shows both responses, the right recurrent laryngeal nerve (upper) and the brain stem (lower). (Continued on page 172.)

curs, and the new waves P_0, N_0 appear. At No.30, even the P_1-N_1 component disappears, and only the P_0-N_0 component remains. From No.37 to No.53, P_0-N_0 latency also elongates, and from No.55, the LBSR becomes almost flat.

Experiment III: Origin of the Earlier Components of LBSR

In this part of the study, the origin of the earlier components was investigated by displacing the recording electrode and by cutting the ipsilateral vagus nerve just above the nodose ganglion. Ventilation time was 30/min and the ventilation volume was changed to maintain the expired gas within a normal range. (Fukuhara, 1986). The ventilatory status was controlled within 16.0–18.0 for FeO_2 and 2.0–3.5 for $FeCO_2$ by monitoring the expired gas analyzer. When the location of the recording electrode was changed, the LBSR was also changed.

When the negative recording electrode was moved to the vicinity of the right tympanic bulla from the III cervical vertebra, earlier components of $P_1-N_1-P_2$ showed an inversion of polarity, and a two-fold increase in amplitude, whereas the later components became obscure (Figure 16-7). On the contrary, such a change did not occur when the positive recording electrode was moved to the level of both bullae (Figure 16-8). A tendency for a reduction of the N_1-P_2 components was seen only when the positive recording electrode was moved to the vicinity of the left bulla, away from the right superior laryngeal nerve being stimulated (Figure 16-8C). When the posi-

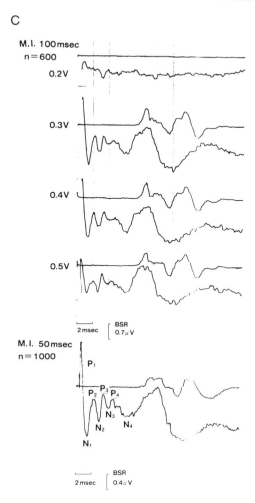

Figure 16-2 (*continued*).

tive recording electrode was displaced to the level of the jugular foramen, a great change occurred . When the positive recording electrode was displaced to the vicinity of the right bulla, $P_1-N_1-P_2$ components increased to more than twice the value at other locations. The latter were in the midposition of both jugular foramina and the vicinity of the left jugular foramen (Figure 16-9A-C). As the electrode was placed adjacent to the nodose ganglion, $P_1-N_1-P_2$ components became even greater (Figure 16-9D). Finally, with the exception of P_1-N_1, later components disappeared after section of the vagus nerve just above the nodose ganglion, although the location of the positive recording electrode was the same as in B (Figure 16-9B).

Experiment IV: Effect of Removing the Cerebellum

The effect on LBSR of removing the cerebellum was studied. The cerebellum was removed with the dorsal approach (Figure 16-10). Ventilatory status was controlled as in experiment III.

LBSR before cerebellum removal is shown in Figure 16-10A. In the bottom row, components after P_3 disappeared at subthreshold stimulation as in experiment I. After cerebellum removal, the reflex potential of the recurrent laryngeal nerve showed an approximately 1 ms delay of latency (Figure 16-10B). Corresponding with this phenomenon, each component of LBSR also showed some delay. The greatest delay for each component was about 1 ms in the N_4 component. This delay value for the N_4 component is the

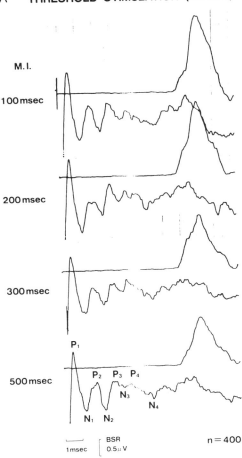

A THRESHOLD STIMULATION (0.165V)

M.I.

100 msec

200 msec

300 msec

500 msec

P_1

P_2 P_3 P_4

N_3

N_4

N_1 N_2

BSR $n = 400$

1 msec 0.5 μV

Figure 16-3. *LBSR obtained by changing the stimulus interval while the stimulus voltage was kept constant.* *(Continued on page 174.)*

same as that of the recurrent laryngeal nerve. In spite of the delay
phenomenon in both LBSR and
the recurrent laryngeal nerve, the
fundamental pattern of LBSR
never changed.

DISCUSSION

LBSR was unaffected by
changes in the polarity of electrical stimulation. Thus, we can as-
sume that these wave forms contained no electrical artifacts. LBSR
was stable with changes of
stimulus.

In the second series of experiments, LBSR demonstrated a sequential response which showed
elongation of latency and disappearance of the response in the
later component. Consequently, it
can be assumed that the later
component is damaged sooner
than the earlier component. As the
circulatory condition was not monitored in these experiments, it cannot be determined whether these
results are due to changes in
respiratory status or to some other
combination of factors.

The remarkable increase of the
$P_1-N_1-P_2$ components after displacement of the positive recording electrode adjacent to the
vagus nerve and the remarkably
inverted increase of these components with displacement of the
negative electrode show that the
earlier $P_1-N_1-P_2$ components
must be generated near the ipsilateral vagus nerve. Furthermore,
the fact that the earlier components never disappear after the
vagus nerve is cut proves that the
earlier $P_1-N_1-P_2$ components are
generated by the afferent vagus

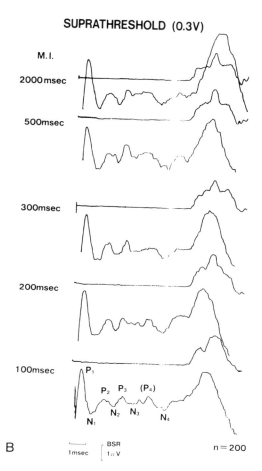

Figure 16-3 *(continued)*.

nerve itself. Consequently, the P_2–N_2–P_3 components must be due to the ipsilateral field potentials evoked by the nucleus solitarius, which is known to be the first input nucleus of the afferent laryngeal vagus nerve (Kalia and Mesulam, 1980). The N_2 latency of LBSR conforms well to the data of the near field recordings by microelectrodes (Porter, 1963; Biscoe and Sampson, 1970a; Sessle, 1973a; Sessle, 1973b; Lucier and Sessle, 1981). The response latency in the vicinity of the nucleus solitarius with stimulation of the ipsilateral superior laryngeal nerve was found by Porter (1963) to be about 2.5 ms, by Biscoe and Sampson (1970b) to be 1.3–2.0 ms and by Sessle (1973a) to have a mean value of 3.5 ms.

The response latency in the nodose ganglion by the antidromic stimulation to the ipsilateral solitary tract nucleus was less than 2.5 ms (Sessle, 1973a), and 1.0–1.5 ms (Lucier and Sessle, 1981). The response latency in the nodose ganglion by orthodromic stimulation of the ipsilateral superior laryngeal nerve was 1.1 ± 0.9 ms (Lucier and Sessle, 1981).

The last negative N_4 component is thought to be due to the ipsilateral field potential evoked by the nucleus ambiguus. This is known as the last output nucleus to the laryngeal and pharyngeal effectors (Kalia and Mesulam, 1980; Yoshida, Miyazaki, Hirano, Shin, and Kanaseki, 1982; Mitsumasu, 1984). The response delay of 1.5–2.0 ms from the peak of the N_4 component to the onset of the laryngeal nerve reflex shows good conformance with the electrophysiological data reported by

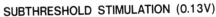

SUBTHRESHOLD STIMULATION (0.13V)

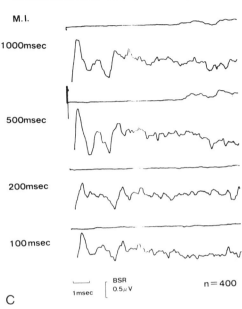

M.I.

1000msec

500msec

200msec

100msec

C

1msec BSR 0.5μV n = 400

Figure 16-3 (*continued*).

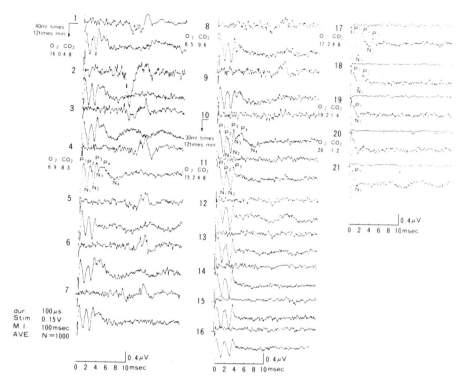

Figure 16-4. *The effect of hypoventilation on LBSR. The upper trace of each left-hand number shows the action potentials of the recurrent laryngeal nerve, and the lower trace LBSR. The number means the sequential time course.*

Porter (1963) and Delgado-Garcia, Lopez-Barneo, Serra, and Gonzalez-Baron, (1983). They reported that the antidromic latency with stimulation of the vagus nerve in the vicinity of the nucleus ambiguus was about 2 ms.

It can be deduced from this that the P_3–N_3–P_4 component must originate in the field potential of interposed neurons in the reticular formation.

However, the essential question remains unsolved: Does LBSR reflect only the summed field potential of the ipsilateral brain stem response to stimulation of the superior laryngeal nerve? Sessle (1973a) reported that he failed to find any neurons in the solitary tract nucleus that could be excited by contralateral superior laryngeal nerve stimulation. This means that only ipsilateral field potentials of the solitary tract nucleus will be recorded in LBSR. Kirchner and Suzuki (1968) and Suzuki and Sasaki (1976) also reported crossed laryngeal reflexes in cats. These occurred only when the stimulus voltage exceeded 0.5 V, which is twice as strong as threshold stimulation. The synaptic delay of the crossed reflex as compared to the ipsilateral reflex is more than 3 ms. Thus, even if the crossed reflex may have occurred in the LBSR, the contralateral component due to the contralateral nucleus ambiguus must have been superimposed in the recurrent laryngeal nerve potentials. Consequently, the laryngeal brain stem responses recorded here are interpreted as reflecting the field potential of the ipsilaterally evoked brain stem response.

The etiological basis of the reflex delay after removal of the cerebellum is unknown. However, it can be said that a critical difference is unlikely to occur with removal of the cerebellum because the fundamental pattern of the LBSR never changes.

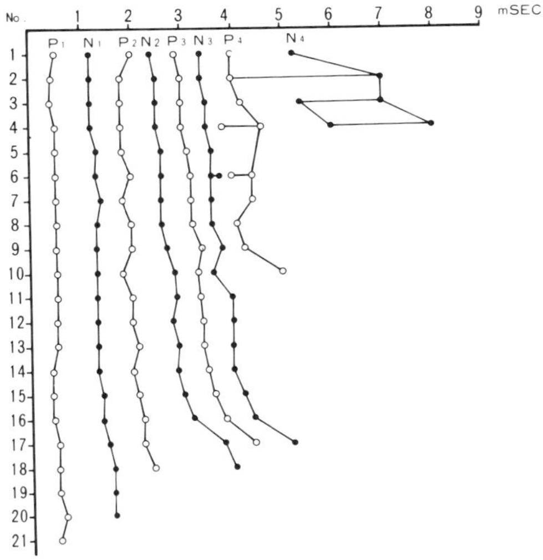

Figure 16-5. *Analysis data of the latency distribution shown in Figure 16-4.*

SUMMARY

The purpose of this research was to complete an electrophysiological study of the synaptic circuit of the laryngeal reflex, using the average method with a far field recording technique. A series of four interrelated experiments led to the following conclusions:

1. LBSR evoked by the laryngeal reflex was recorded by the averaging method, locating the recording electrodes on either side of the brainstem.

2. LBSR was composed of four positive waves termed P_1–P_4, and four negative waves termed N_1–N_4. The following latencies were identified:

P_1, 0.5–1 ms
P_2, 1.6–2.3 ms

P_3, 2.8–3.2 ms

P_4 latency changed according to the stimulus conditions

N_1, 1.2–1.3 ms

N_2, 2.4–2.7 ms

N_3, 3.4–3.6 ms

N_4, 5–5.5 ms

3. LBSR was stable during changes of the stimulus with only one exception: the N_4 component became obscure with sub-threshold stimulation.

4. LBSR appeared to be a sequential response that showed elongation of latency and disappearance of the response in the later component.

5. $P_1–N_1–P_2$ components seemed to be evoked by the afferent vagus nerve, $P_2–N_2–P_3$ components by the nucleus of the tractus solitarius, and N_4 by the nucleus ambiguus.

6. A latency delay in both the recurrent laryngeal nerve reflex and LBSR was observed as a result of removing the cerebellum. In particular, the N_4 component was delayed for about 1 ms which was the same as that of the laryngeal nerve reflex.

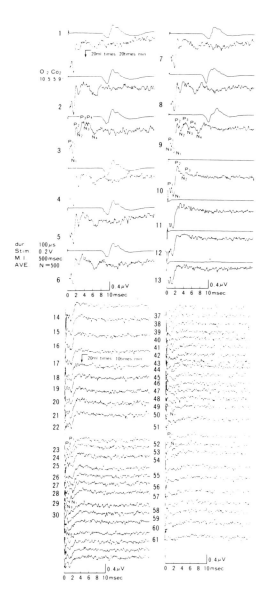

Figure 16-6. *Another case showing effects of hypoventilation.*

神
経
喉
頭
科
学

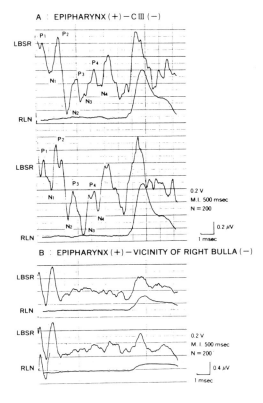

Figure 16-7. *By displacement of the negative recording electrode to the vicinity of the right tympanic bulla (B) from the III cervical vertebra (A), earlier components of P_1–N_1–P_2 showed an inversion of polarity and an almost two-fold increase in amplitude. Later components are obscure.*

神経喉頭科学

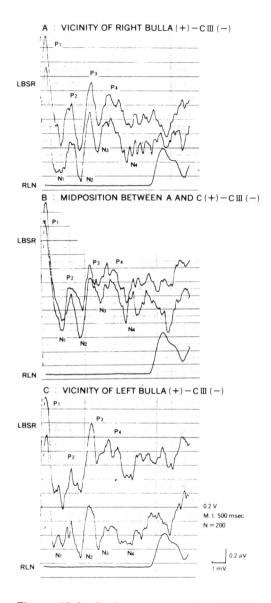

Figure 16-8. *A change as great as that in Figure 16-7 does not occur when the positive recording electrode is displaced to the level of both bullae.*

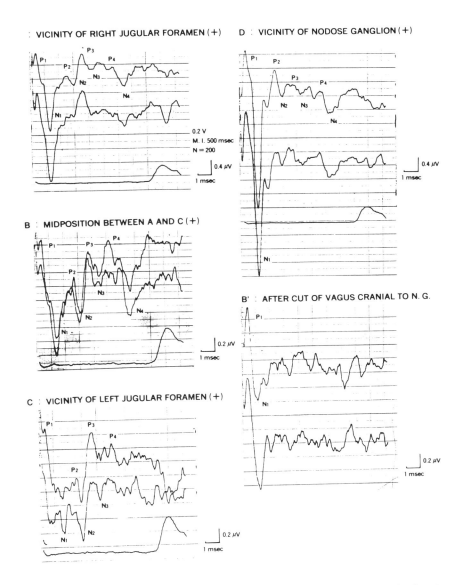

A : VICINITY OF RIGHT JUGULAR FORAMEN (+)

P₁ P₂ P₃ P₄ N₂ N₃ N₄ N₁

0.2 V
M. I. 500 msec
N = 200

0.4 μV
1 msec

D : VICINITY OF NODOSE GANGLION (+)

P₁ P₂ P₃ P₄ N₂ N₃ N₄ N₁

0.4 μV
1 msec

B : MIDPOSITION BETWEEN A AND C (+)

P₁ P₃ P₄ P₂ N₃ N₄ N₂ N₁

0.2 μV
1 msec

B' : AFTER CUT OF VAGUS CRANIAL TO N. G.

P₁ N₁

0.2 μV
1 msec

C : VICINITY OF LEFT JUGULAR FORAMEN (+)

P₁ P₃ P₄ P₂ N₃ N₂ N₁

0.2 μV
1 msec

Figure 16-9. *The positive recording electrode was displaced to the level of the jugular foramina, in the vicinity of the right bulla (A), in the midposition of both jugular foramina (B), and in the vicinity of the left jugular foramen (C). The positive electrode was adjacent to the nodose ganglion (D). B′ shows the data obtained after cutting the vagus nerve just above the nodose ganglion. The location of the positive recording electrode was unchanged from B.*

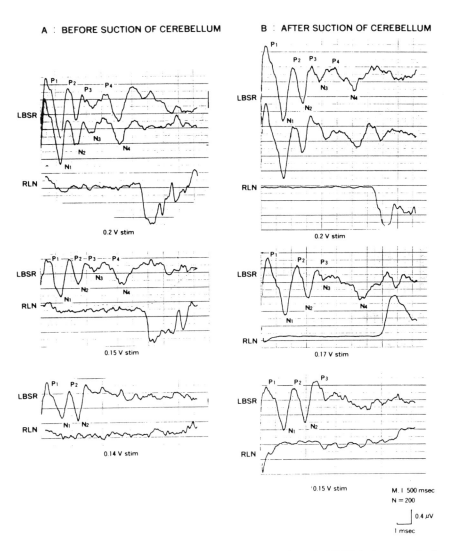

Figure 16-10. *The effect of cerebellar removal by suction. A: LBSR before cerebellum removal. B: LBSR after cerebellum removal.*

REFERENCES

Biscoe, T.J., and Sampson, S.R. (1970a). Field potentials evoked in the brain stem of the cat by stimulation of the carotid sinus, glossopharyngeal, aortic and superior laryngeal nerves. *J Physiol, 209*, 341–358.

Biscoe, T.J., and Sampson, S.R. (1970b). Responses of cells in the brain stem of the cat to stimulation of the sinus, glossopharyngeal, aortic and superior laryngeal nerves. *J Physiol, 209*, 359–373.

Delgado-Garcia, J.M., Lopez-Barneo, J., Serra, R., and Gonzalez-Baron, S. (1983). Electrophysiological and functional identification of different neuronal types within the nucleus ambiguus. *Brain Res, 277*, 231–240.

Fukuhara, T. (1986). *Application of the expired gas analyzer to physiological and pharmacological studies.* Tokyo: Sanei.

Kirchner, J.A., and Suzuki, M. (1968). Laryngeal reflexes and vocal production. *Ann NY Acad Sci, 155*, 98–109.

Kalia, M., and Mesulam, M. (1980). Brain stem projections of sensory and motor components of the vagus complex in the cat: II. Laryngeal, tracheobronchial, pulmonary, cardiac, and gastrointestinal branches. *J Comp Neuro, 193*, 467–508.

Lucier, G.E., and Sessle, B.J. (1981). Presynaptic excitability changes induced in the solitary tract endings of laryngeal primary afferents by stimulation of nucleus Raphe Magnus and locus Coeruleus. *Neurosci Lett 26*, 221–226.

Mitsumasu, T. (1984). Afferent projections to the nucleus ambiguus in the cats. *Otologia Fukuoka 30*, 1106–1134.

Porter, R. (1963). Unit responses evoked in the medulla oblongata by vagus nerve stimulation. *J Physiol, 168*, 717–735.

Sessle, B.J. (1973a). Excitatory and inhibitory inputs to single neurons in the solitary tract nucleus and adjacent reticular formation. *Brain Res, 53*, 319–331.

Sessle, B.J. (1973b). Presynaptic excitability changes induced in single laryngeal primary afferent fibers. *Brain Res, 53*, 333–342.

Suzuki, M., and Sasaki, C.T. (1976). Initiation of reflex glottic closure. *Ann Otol Rhinol Laryngol, 85*, 382–386.

Yoshida, Y., Miyazaki, T., Hirano, M., Shin, T., and Kanaseki, T. (1982). Arrangement of motoneurons innervating the intrinsic laryngeal muscles of cats as demonstrated by horseradish peroxidase. *Acta Otolaryngol (Stockh), 94*, 329–334.

CHAPTER 17

Response of the Human Larynx to Auditory Stimulation

Jiro UDAKA,
Hiroyuki KANETAKA
and Yasuo KOIKE

In mammals, the larynx responds promptly to various types of external stimulation for purposes of protection and phonation. This is especially true of human speech, in which the auditory system influences laryngeal function through an elaborate reflex mechanism. Suzuki and Sasaki (1977) and others (Jen and Suga, 1976; Yonovitz and Lozar, 1983) have demonstrated the existence, in the mammalian larynx, of an auditory-laryngeal reflex with short latency. With regard to the human larynx, Baer (1979) reported that during sustained phonation, an auditory stimulus changed the fundamental frequency level. Sapir, McClean, and Larson (1983) reported that in experiments similar to those of Baer, cricothyroid muscle activity changed before the fundamental frequency level.

In this study, we examined the influence of the auditory system on human laryngeal control by measuring EMG changes in the intrinsic laryngeal muscles.

METHODS

Subjects

Eleven healthy subjects with no abnormality of speech participated in this investigation. The subjects were 24 to 61 years of age (average, 37 years). Nine were men and two were women.

Data Aquisition and Equipment

Each subject was shown the monitor screen of a phonolaryngograph (Rion SH-01), and asked to sustain phonation at constant pitch and comfortable loudness. During phonation, the subject received repeated auditory click stimuli. The fundamental frequency and intensity levels of phonation were recorded through a microphone and displayed on the monitor screen. Irregular click stimuli (duration, 90 ms, once per s average) were generated by an auditory stimulator (NEC-Sanei 3G26) and delivered to both ears through a headphone. Pretracheal sounds were recorded through a contact microphone attached to the anterior neck just below the cricoid cartilage. EMG activity of one or both cricothyroid (CT) and lateral cricoarytenoid (LCA) muscles was recorded with stainless wire bipolar hooked electrodes (0.1 mm thick) inserted percutaneously. The signal was amplified by an electromyograph (Medelec MS6, Filter 16Hz-3.2kHz). Data were stored in an FM data recorder (Teac MS-30) (Figure 17-1).

Data Analysis and Equipment

The EMG signal was rectified and averaged with the triggered pulse of clicks by a signal processor (NEC-Sanei 7T07) to determine how the muscle activity was changed by auditory stimulation. For clarification of the response, the EMG signal was smoothed by digital filtration of the signal processor, and the latency between stimulus and maximum amplitude of the wave was measured. Only the alternating component (AC) of the wave was recorded. To calculate its change, the fundamental frequency was picked out from the pretracheal sound in

some cases, and averaged in the same manner as the EMG signal. The number of points averaged was 80 for EMG signals, and 40 for pretracheal sounds (Figure 17-2).

Conditions of the Experiment

Some subjects were asked to sustain phonation at various pitches while receiving auditory clicks of various intensities to determine the conditions under which reactions were greatest. One subject was retested under the same conditions on another day to confirm the reliability of the recording. Reactions without phonation, and during stimulation of sensory nerves other than the auditory, were also examined. Finally, all subjects were reexamined for latencies under the conditions determined in the first test to be most suitable.

RESULTS

Experiment 1

Subject 8 was asked to sustain phonation at 420 Hz and received various loudness levels (90, 70, 50, and 30 dB) of auditory clicks to determine a suitable auditory stimulus for producing a laryngeal response. At a click sound level of 90 dB, the activity of the left CT showed maximum amplitude after about 30 ms. At 70 dB, the amplitude was lower, but the response was similar. No response was recognized with stimuli of 50 and 30 dB (Figure 17-3).

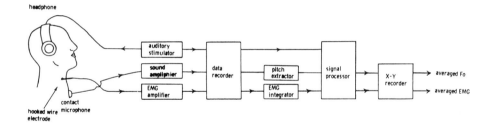

Figure 17-1. *Block diagram of experimental arrangement.*

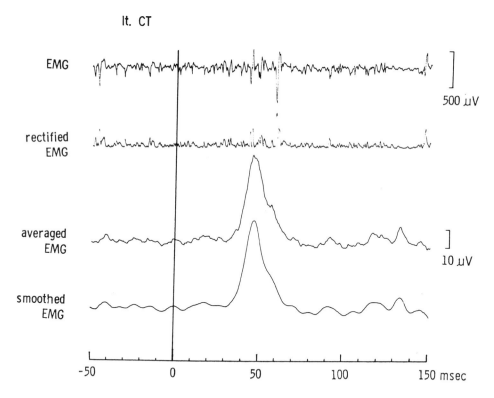

Figure 17-2. *EMG signal of subject 5 processed from top to bottom. O: auditory stimulus point. CT: cricothyroid muscle.*

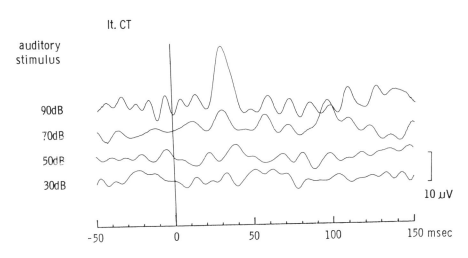

Figure 17-3. *EMG signal of subject 8 on auditory stimulus at various intensities.*

Experiment 2

For confirmation of the reliability of the method, the average responses of the left CT to 40 stimulations at two different times (A-1 and A-2) were determined in subject 7 . Similar response waves were observed in the two tests. In addition, when this subject was asked to phonate under the same conditions as before, almost the same latency was observed, but the maximum amplitude was different the second time (B) (Figure 17-4).

Experiment 3

Subject 8 was asked to sustain phonation not only at high pitch (420 Hz), but also at intermediate (155 Hz), and low (100 Hz) pitches, while receiving auditory stimulation at 90 dB. At the intermediate pitch of phonation, the amplitude of the response wave was smaller, but the latency was similar to that at high pitch. This response was not recognized during low pitch phonation (Figure 17-5).

Experiment 4

Subject 7 also received auditory stimulation without phonation when his EMG activity was increased in preparation for phonation. Results showed that regardless of the presence or absence of phonation, whenever muscle activity increased, the EMG latency was the same (Figure 17-6).

Experiment 5

Subject 11 was asked to sustain high pitch phonation while receiving 40 electrical stimuli (voltage 40 V, duration 0.2 ms) to the right or left supraorbital nerve, which was selected as another cranial sensory nerve instead of the auditory nerve. The EMG signals of the left CT were averaged. The latency was much delayed, but EMG acti-

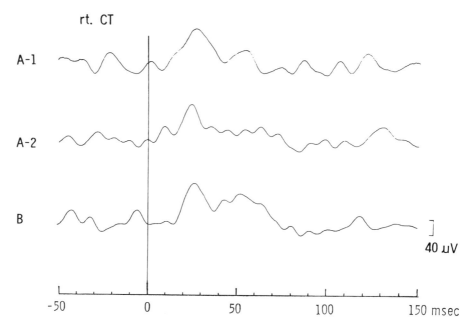

Figure 17-4. *EMG signal of subject 7 at different times.*

vity increased during auditory nerve stimulation. A latency difference was observed with stimulation of the right and left supraorbital nerves (Figure 17-7). In the LCA, phenomena analogous to those seen in experiments 1 through 5 were observed.

Experiment 6

From the results of these preliminary experiments, we selected 90 dB as the standard condition of auditory stimulation during high pitch phonation. With these conditions, all subjects showed increased EMG activity with some latency. The latency to the maximum amplitude in five subjects was 22 to 31 ms (mean = 26.1 ms) in the right CT; 20 to 30.5 ms

(mean = 26.3 ms) in the left CT; 42 to 49 ms (mean = 45.2 ms) in the right LCA; and 44 to 49 ms (mean = 47 ms) in the left LCA (Table 17-1). Figure 17-8 shows the overlap of EMG signals of each muscle. Using the averaging process, we obtained a fairly clear value for the latency to the maximum amplitude, but not the time of initiation of the response.

Typical Case

Results on subject 5 are given as examples of the EMG signals recorded from the four muscles (Figure 17-9). This healthy man of 29 years, 178 cm height, was asked to sustain phonation at 350 Hz while receiving auditory stimuli of 90 dB to both ears. Figure 17-9

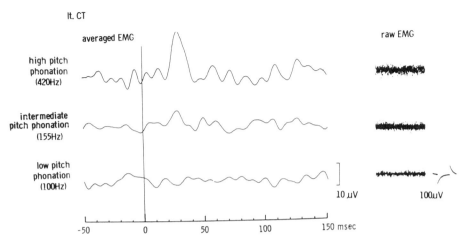

Figure 17-5. *EMG signal of subject 8 at various pitches of phonation.*

shows changes in the fundamental frequency level, and in the EMG signals from the right CT, left CT, right LCA, and left LCA. The fundamental frequency began to increase after about 60 ms and reached the highest level, about 3 Hz, approximately 100 ms after auditory stimulation. Preceding that, the EMG activity of the right CT increased and its peak showed a latency time of about 31 ms. A similar change in the EMG of the left CT was observed. However, the reaction of the LCA began later. The latency time of the peak EMG activity in the right LCA was about 43 ms, and that of left was about 46 ms, (3 ms later than that of the right).

Next, to clarify the beginning of the reaction, each raw EMG wave was displayed continuously at higher magnification (Figure 17-10). In each wave, some time after auditory stimulation, the motor unit potentials (MUPs) recruited and increased in number. The MUP amplitude itself also became larger than before stimulation. The latency times differed slightly, the shortest being only about 10 ms. After recruitment, the EMG activity showed suppression 40 to 60 ms after auditory stimulation in the I, II and III raw EMG waves. The duration of suppression was 30 to 50 ms. The MUP of the left LCA also showed recruitment after stimulation. Its latency time, however, was much longer than that of the CT. Even the shortest latency time was about 20 ms (Figure 17-11).

DISCUSSION

Experiment 1 showed that auditory stimulation during phonation increased the EMG activity of the intrinsic laryngeal muscles: the amplitude increased with increasing intensity of stimulation. The latency from the time of the stimulus to that of maximum amplitude

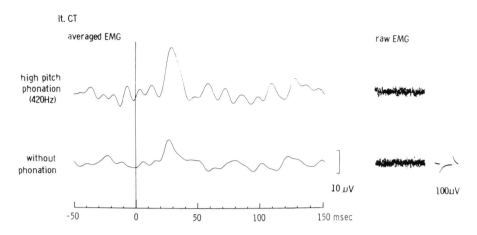

Figure 17-6. *EMG signal of subject 7 with high pitch phonation and without phonation.*

was almost the same at different intensities of stimulation. Sapir and colleagues (1983) reported that the magnitude of reaction was related to the intensity of auditory stimulation, and that a reaction was observed when the level of auditory stimulation was more than 45 dB.

In experiment 2, repetition of the same stimulus intensity in the same subject resulted in the same change in EMG activity. Thus, this change is probably nonhabitual, reproducible, and consistent in humans.

Experiment 3 showed that the higher the pitch of sustained phonation, the larger the reaction.

Experiment 4 indicated that the latency time was almost the same during increased muscle activity, regardless of phonation. This means that the magnitude of the reaction was related to the EMG activity rather than to the pitch of phonation. In other words, the reaction was so small that it was clearly observed only under high-

pitch phonation, when an MUP of larger amplitude participated according to the size principle (Henneman, Somjen, and Carpenter, 1965). As shown in animals, (Jen and Suga, 1976; Suzuki and Sasaki, 1977; Yonovitz and Lozar, 1983), if the stimulus is applied to the superior or recurrent laryngeal nerve, the EMG response is clearer.

In experiment 5, a similar increase in EMG activity with different latency was observed during stimulation of a sensory nerve unrelated to phonation, and the phenomenon was also observed in the LCAs. Latency times differed with stimulation of the right and left supraorbital nerves. This phenomenon is similar to the "synaptic delay" described by Kirchner and Suzuki (1968) in the recurrent laryngeal nerve response induced by stimulation of the internal branch of the superior laryngeal nerve in cats. It is probably due to the primitive nature of the glottic closure reaction, and not involved

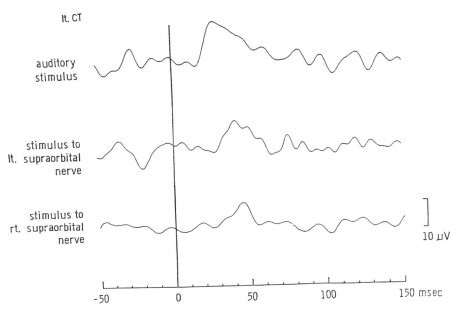

Figure 17-7. *EMG signals of subject 11 on various stimuli.*

with a more direct control of the phonation such as pitch, as Sapir and colleagues (1983) suggested. But further investigations are needed on this point.

Intensive auditory stimulation during high pitch phonation produced a similar reaction in all subjects. In most subjects, there was a slight difference in the latency times of the maximum amplitudes of the EMG in the CTs, which are controlled by the superior laryngeal nerve, but in subjects 5, 8, and 9 there was scarcely any difference between the two muscles. In other words, there was a difference not within each subject, but among subjects. On the other hand, some difference was found between the latencies of the right and left LCAs, which were controlled by the recurrent laryngeal nerve. The latencies of the left and right LCAs were similar in subject 1, but that of the right one was less than that of the left by 2 ms in subject 2, 3 ms in subjects 3 and 5, and 1.5 ms in subject 4. In all cases, the latency of the CT was less than that of the LCA. Average values showed that both CTs reacted first, at almost the same time, about 26 ms after stimulation, followed by the right LCA about 20 ms later, and then the left LCA about 2 ms later.

In subject 5, in whom the reactions of four muscles were recorded simultaneously, both CTs reacted first, about 31 ms after auditory stimulation, followed by the right LCA about 12 ms later, and finally the left LCA about 3 ms later. It is interesting that the two CTs had almost the same laten-

TABLE 17-1.
Latencies (in milliseconds) of the maximum amplitude in all the subjects

No.	Sex	Age	Cricothyroid m. Right	Cricothyroid m. Left	Lateral Cricoarytenoid m. Right	Lateral Cricoarytenoid m. Left
1	F	55			49.0	48.5
2	M	61			42.0	44.0
3	M	26			44.5	47.5
4	M	30			47.5	49.0
5	M	26	31.0	30.5	43.0	46.0
6	M	24	24.0			
7	M	58	25.0			
8	M	24	28.5	28.5		
9	M	27	22.0	23.0		
10	M	26		20.0		
11	F	50		29.5		
Average		37	26.1	26.3	45.2	47.0

cies, but that the right and left LCAs had different latencies. Atkins (1973) reported that the difference in electrical conduction times of the right and left recurrent laryngeal nerves from their origin in the vagus nerve (approximately 2.5 cm below the cricoid) to the thyroarytenoid muscle was about 2 ms. Similarly, Sato (1978) found that the difference between the right and left in electrical conduction times was 2 to 3 ms. The difference between latencies of the right and left auditory-laryngeal tracts that we observed was almost the same as the difference in the conduction times of only the peripheral portions of the right and left recurrent laryngeal nerves. Therefore, the main reason for the difference in the latencies on the two sides seems to be the difference in lengths of the right and left recurrent laryngeal nerves. It has been hypothesized (Shin and

Rabuzzi, 1971) that the difference in lengths of the right and left recurrent laryngeal nerves is compensated for by a difference in their conduction velocities, and that both intrinsic laryngeal muscles contract in response to stimuli from the central nervous system at almost the same time. However, from our 50 results this was not the case. Atkins (1973) reported that the left and right recurrent laryngeal nerves of a person of 180 cm height differ by about 15 cm in length. Supposing that both recurrent laryngeal nerves have the same conduction velocity, applying the difference in the latencies of the left and right LCAs of about 3 ms that we observed here, the conduction velocity can be calculated to be about 50 m/s, which seems appropriate. Although the CT and LCA are both intrinsic laryngeal muscles, their latencies to the maximum amplitude differed by more than 10 ms, and they seemed to contract independently. Reported times from electrical activation of intrinsic laryngeal muscles to actual muscle activation (contraction time) observed in animals on electrical stimulation and determined in humans by the cross correlation method (Martensson and Skoglund, 1964; Atkinson, 1978; Sato, Yanohara, Takenouchi, Suzuki, Hisa, and Hyuga, 1982) are indicated in Table 17-2. For example, Sato and colleagues (1982) reported that in dogs, the contraction time of the CT was 38 ms, and that of the LCA was 20 ms. The latency to the maximum amplitude of the CT was shorter than that of the LCA and the contraction time of the former was longer than that of the latter. The time from the beginning of auditory stimulation to the actual time of muscle activation was almost the same for the four muscles. Therefore, these four muscles are thought to work in cooperation. The time lag of about 30 ms between the appearance of actual muscle activity and the change of fundamental frequency is considered to be due to the effects of other factors, for example, the effect of an antagonistic muscle such as the posterior cricoarytenoid muscle, or lung compliance. In any case, at least 100 ms would be required for the actual change in form of the vocal fold.

A fairly clear value for the maximum amplitude was obtained by averaging the EMG signals, but the exact time of the beginning of the reaction was not clear. In the EMG signal of subject 5, in whom the reaction appeared greatest, we examined the record in detail

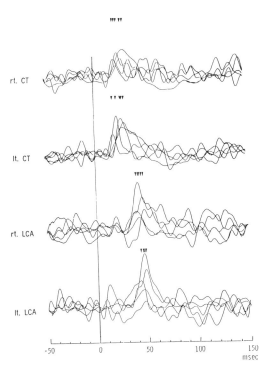

Figure 17-8. *Over-lapped EMG signals of each muscle. LCA: lateral cricoarytenoid muscle. →: point of maximum amplitude.*

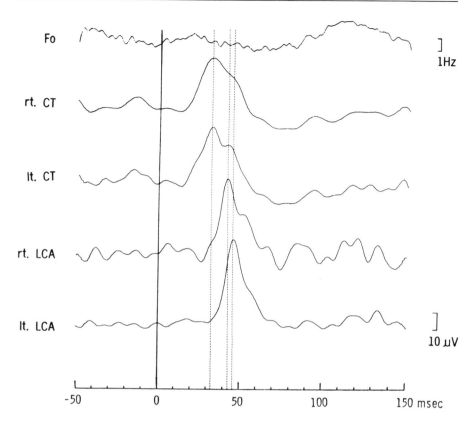

Figure 17-9. F_0 and EMG signals of four muscles of subject 5. F_0: fundamental frequency.

to determine the beginning of the latency (short latency) when the reaction began. The shortest latency was about 10 ms in the raw EMG waves of the CT. Sapir and colleagues (1983) reported that Cummings had found that the length of the superior laryngeal nerve from the ambiguus nucleus to the CT was at least 10 ms. Applying the value for the conduction velocity reported by Ogura and Lam (1953) of 50 m/s, the conduction time of the superior laryngeal nerve was calculated to be about 2 ms. Supposing that conduction

through the end plate and electrical excitation of the CT require about 1 ms, and the reaction time from auditory stimulation to the cochlear nucleus requires about 3 ms, the conduction time from the cochlear nucleus to the ambiguus nucleus should be a few ms. Therefore, this reaction is considered to be a "reflex" that takes place at the brain stem level, unrelated to the cerebrum.

On the other hand, the MUP is thought by some to be recruited after stimulation of the LCA, as in the CT. For example, the EMG sig-

It. CT

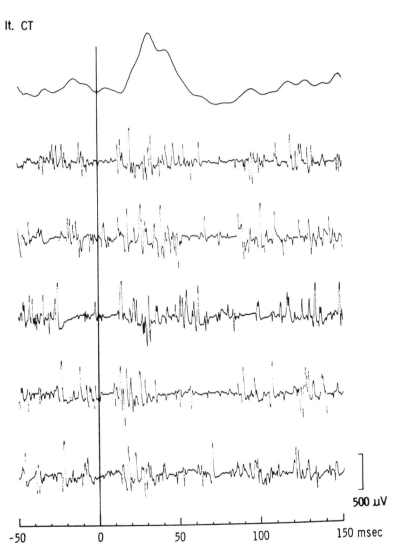

Figure 17-10. *Averaged and raw EMG signals of the left CT of subject 5.*

195

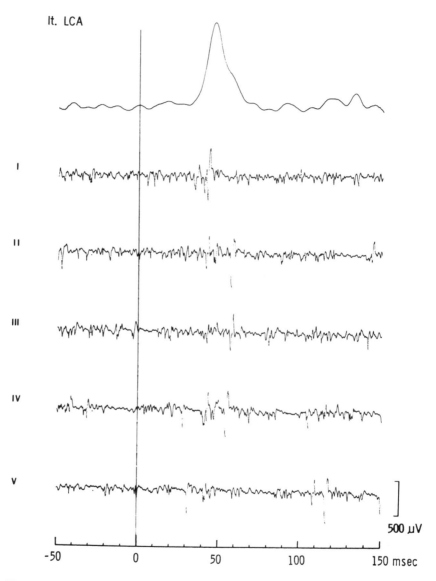

Figure 17-11. *Averaged and raw EMG signals of the left LCA of subject 5.*

TABLE 17-2.
Reported contraction times.

	CT	LCA	Subjects
Martensson and Skoglund (1964)	35 ms	16 ms	dogs
Atkinson (1978)	40 ms	15 ms	humans (estimating value)
Sato et al. (1982)	38 ms	21 ms	dogs

nal of the left LCA of this subject is seen in Figure 17-11, but its shortest latency was longer by at least 20 ms than that of the CT. According to Krmpotic (1958), the right recurrent laryngeal nerve is 32.2 cm long and the left one is an average of 42.6 cm long from the nucleus ambiguus to the peripheral portion. Applying the value for the conduction velocity of 50 m/sec which we calculated from the difference in the left and right recurrent laryngeal nerves, conduction of a stimulus from the nucleus ambiguus to the peripheral portion requires about 6 ms in the left and about 8 ms in the right recurrent laryngeal nerve. In this subject, the reaction time from the cochlear nucleus to the nucleus ambiguus was about 10 ms, which was rather short, but much longer than that of the superior laryngeal nerve, which was a few ms. This means that the laryngeal reflex in response to auditory stimulation was elicited in the brain stem through the superior laryngeal nerve and recurrent laryngeal nerve separately. However, as the conduction velocity and effects of other factors were uncertain in this experiment, further studies are needed on this problem.

At present, this is the only method available for determining the relation between the larynx and the sensory nerves. Further study is required for many problems, such as the maximum amplitude of the EMG response and the mechanism of central control of this phenomenon. In addition, a method suitable for clinical use must be established.

REFERENCES

Atkins, J.P., Jr. (1973). An electromyographic study of recurrent laryngeal nerve conduction and its clinical applications. *Laryngoscope, 83,* 796–807.

Atkinson, J.E. (1978). Correlation analysis of the physiological factors controlling fundamental voice frequency. *J Acoust Soc Am, 63,* 211–222.

Baer, T. (1979). Reflex activation of laryngeal muscles by sudden induced subglottal pressure changes. *J Acoust Soc Am, 63,* 1271–1275.

Henneman, E., Somjen, G., and Carpenter, D.O. (1965). Functional significance of cell size in spinal motoneurons. *J Neurophysiol, 28,* 560–580.

Jen, P.H.S., and Suga, K.N. (1976). Coordinated activity of middle-ear and laryngeal muscles in echolocating bats. *Science, 191,* 950–952.

Kirchner, J.A., and Suzuki, K. (1968). Laryngeal reflexes and voice production. *Ann NY Acad Sci, 155,* 98–109.

Krmpotic, J. (1958). Anatomisch-histologische und funkutionelle Verhältnisse des rechten und des linken Nervus recurrens mit Rucksicht auf die Geschwindingkeit der Impulsleitung bei einer Ursprungsanomalie der rechten Schlüsselbeinarterie. *Arch fur Ohr kehl Heilkunde, 173,* 490–496.

Mårtensson, A., and Skoglund, C.R. (1964). Contraction properties of intrinsic laryngeal muscles. *Acta Physiol Scand, 60,* 318–336.

Ogura, J.H., and Lam, L.R. (1953). Anatomical and physiological correlation on stimulating the human superior laryngeal nerve. *Laryngoscope, 63,* 947–959.

Sapir, S., McClean, M.D., and Larson, C.R. (1983). Human laryngeal responses to auditory stimulation. *J Acoust Soc Am, 73,* 315–321.

Sato, F., Yanohara, K., Takenouchi, S., Suzuki, Y., Hisa, Y., and Hyuga, M. (1982). Mechanical properties of the laryngeal muscles and biomechanics of the glottis in the dog. *J Otolaryngol Jpn, 85,* 951–956.

Sato, I. (1978). Evoked electromyographic test applied for recurrent laryngeal nerve paralysis. *Laryngoscope, 88,* 2022–2031.

Shin, T., and Rabuzzi, D. (1971). Conduction studies of the canine recurrent laryngeal nerve. *Laryngoscope, 81,* 586–596.

Suzuki, M., and Sasaki, C.T. (1977). Effect of various sensory stimuli on reflex laryngeal adduction. *Ann Otol, 86,* 30–36.

Yonovitz, A., and Lozar, J. (1983). The acoustic cricothyroid response in the rat. *J Auditory Res, 23,* 63–71.

PART 4

Muscle Behavior

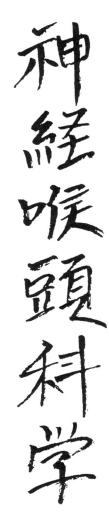

CHAPTER 18

Laryngeal Articulatory Adjustments in Terms of EMG

Hajime HIROSE

Electromyographic (EMG) approaches to laryngeal physiology have provided important perspectives for neurolaryngology. In particular, EMG has proved to be very useful for studying laryngeal participation in voice and speech production, one of the most interesting subjects of modern research on laryngeal physiology.

For the past fifteen years, the author's research group has been exploring the role of active laryngeal adjustments during speech production, mainly using EMG techniques often combined with other methods: fiberoptic observation of the larynx, for example.

The purpose of this paper is to present our findings on the laryngeal muscle actions associated with the segmental and suprasegmental (prosodic) controls of speech.

LARYNGEAL MUSCLE ACTIONS IN THE SEGMENTAL CONTROL OF SPEECH

It has been revealed that there is active participation of the intrinsic laryngeal muscles in the control of laryngeal articulatory gestures in terms of glottal adduction-abduction adjustments. Particularly, the posterior cricoarytenoid (PCA), the only abductor of the vocal folds, has been found to play a subtle role in glottal opening gestures, provided that there is simultaneous suppression of the adductor muscles. In other words, the principal mechanism underlying adduction-abduction is reciprocal activation of the adductor and abductor groups of the larynx. Among the adductors, the interarytenoid (INT) most clearly demonstrates a reciprocity with the PCA in terms of the voicing features in different languages, including American English, Japanese, French, and Danish (Hirose, Yoshioka, and Niimi, 1979).

Figure 18-1 shows an example of computer-averaged EMG curves of the five intrinsic laryngeal muscles for two pairs of test words: /teNki/ versus /deNki/ and /seeteN/ versus /seedeN/, embedded in the frame sentence "sore wa _____ desu" (that is _____) and produced by a Japanese speaker. It can be seen that the PCA and the INT show a pattern of reciprocal activation for the voiceless portions of the test utterances and the corresponding INT suppression varies somewhat depending on the phonetic environment. A similar relationship between the PCA and the INT was also revealed in other phonetic conditions, including voiced-voiceless contrasts in utterance-initial and -final positions (Hirose and Gay, 1972; Hirose, Sawashima, and Yoshioka, 1983).

The result of simultaneous recording of laryngeal EMG and

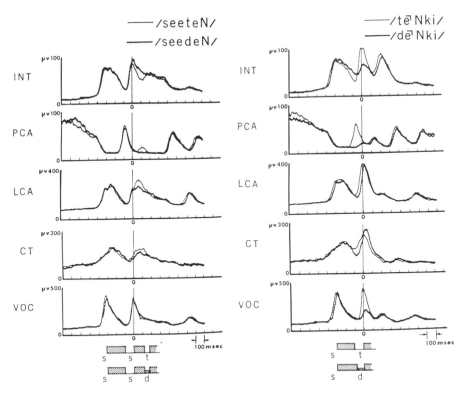

Figure 18-1. *Averaged EMG curves of the five intrinsic laryngeal muscles for test utterances comparing Japanese /t/ and /d/ in word-initial (left) and -medial (right) positions. The line-up point for the averaging was the onset of the vowel after /t/ or /d/.*

the time course of the glottal width as measured using a fiberoptic technique indicated that there is a significant correlation between the peak values of averaged PCA activity and maximum glottai width (Hirose, 1976).

It was also found that, in general, the temporal pattern of PCA activity corresponds to the time course of the glottal aperture change (arytenoid separation) for various voiceless sounds and sound sequences, with an expected time delay.

For example, Figure 18-2 compares the time course of the glottal width (GW), represented by the distance between the tips of the vocal processes, with smoothed integrated EMG curves for the INT and PCA for a single utterance produced by a Japanese speaker. In this example, a test word, /iseH/, embedded in the frame "sore o _____ to yuu" (We call that _____) was used. The envelope of the speech waves (audio) is also compared in the figure. The vertical line indicates the time point of the onset of the vowel [e] following the voiceless sound [s].

It can be seen that the glottis opens for the word-medial voiceless [s]. There is PCA activity approximately 50 ms prior to the glottal opening, the temporal patterns of the two curves being very similar to each other. It can also be seen that there is a decrease in INT activity at the same time as the increase in PCA activity, giving a time curve that is nearly the inverse figure of that for the PCA activity.

The glottal opening gesture and its timing were studied further in more complicated phonetic condi-

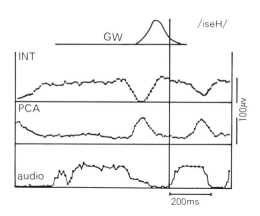

Figure 18-2. *Time curves of the glottal width (GW), smoothed and integrated EMG curves of the INT and PCA, and the audio envelope for a single token of /sore o iseH to yuu/. The vertical line indicates the onset of the vowel /e/ in /iseH/.*

tions for clusters of voiceless obstruents in American English with a combination of EMG, fiberoptics, and transillumination techniques (Yoshioka, Lofqvist, and Hirose, 1981). Here, a comparison was made among three utterance types: "I may scale," "My ace caves," and "I mask aid." As shown in Figure 18-3, two distinct peaks in the PCA activity curves were observed for the [sk] sequence when a word boundary intervened, whereas only one PCA peak was observed for the same sequence without the boundary. The result suggests that each voiceless obstruent with aspiration or frication requires a separate gesture of glottal abduction.

The contribution to the voicing distinction of each intrinsic laryngeal muscle other than the PCA and the INT is not completely understood as yet. When we examine Figure 18-1 further, it is obvious that there are differences in the activity patterns among the three adductors: INT, the lateral cricoarytenoid (LCA), and the thyroarytenoid (VOC). For both LCA and VOC, muscle activity increases at the initiation of each utterance and decreases for word initial consonants, and the degree of reduction is comparable for both voiced and voiceless consonants. The activity increases again after the suppression, apparently for the nuclear vowel fol-

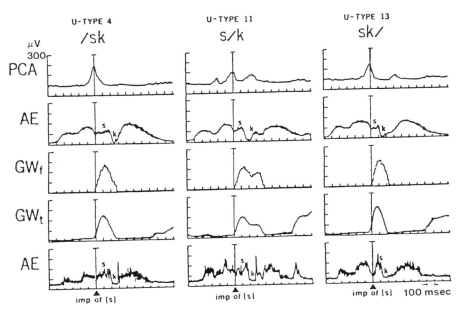

Figure 18-3. *Averaged EMG of the PCA, averaged audio envelopes (AE), representative plots of glottal width using fiberoptics (GW$_f$), corresponding glottograms (GWt) and the audio envelope (AE) for three utterance types: "I may scale" (type 4), "My ace caves" (type 11), and "I mask aid" (type 13).*

lowing the initial consonants.

In the case of the VOC, muscle activity sharply increases after the voiceless consonant, whereas the increase is less marked after the voiced pair. The pattern of LCA activity in terms of the suppression for the initial consonant and the reactivation for the following vowel is essentially the same, regardless of the voicing of the initial consonant. For the consonant segment in the word-medial position, the LCA and VOC curves generally show the pattern of suppression after the activation for the vowel segment of the preceding mora.

It has been reported that the LCA appears to provide supplementary adduction control of the glottis (Hirose, Lisker, and Abramson, 1972; Fischer-Jorgensen and Hirose, 1974; Benguerel, Hirose, Sawashima, and Ushijima, 1978). As the INT action alone does not seem to accomplish the full adduction of the vocal folds (Dixit, 1975; Hirano, 1975), it seems reasonable to consider that the INT provides finer adjustments of the glottal aperture for various speech sounds with the supportive action of the LCA, and possibly with that of the VOC as well, after the larynx is once geared to the so-called speech mode by the activity of all the adductors associated with the suppression of the PCA.

The general pattern of the cricothyroid (CT) activity in Figure 18-1 is characterized by two peaks separated apparently by suppression at the initial consonant of the test words, presumably as a boundary effect in the test utterances. At least in the word-initial position, the suppression is less marked for the voiceless cognate than for the voiced. It may be plausible to consider the relatively high CT activity in the production of a voiceless consonant in certain cases as one possible factor in enhancing voicelessness, as the CT can contribute to the increase in the longitudinal tension of the vocal fold, which may eventually be relevant for eliminating voicing. However, our previous studies have not always confirmed the CT contribution to voicelessness (Kagaya and Hirose, 1975; Hirose and Ushijima, 1978). Thus, the interpretation of the apparently high CT activity in certain consonantal segments is still not understood and remains to be investigated further.

It has been claimed that another dimension independent of the glottal adduction-abduction gesture must also be taken into consideration in the case of laryngeal adjustments with regard to specific phonetic phenomena. Laryngeal control in the production of the Korean forced stop is one example of this type of phenomena, in which a very distinct, sharp activation of the VOC is characteristic, as shown in Figure 18-4 (Hirose, Lee, and Ushijima, 1974; Hirose, 1977). This VOC activity presumably results in an increase in the tension of the vocal fold body, as well as in a constriction of the glottis during or immediately after the articulatory closure. This VOC gesture can be considered a physiological correlate of so-called laryngealization (Hirose and Sawashima, 1981).

A similar type of VOC activation is also found in the case of the Danish "stød" (Figure 18-5). Whether this mode of VOC contraction is necessary for a relatively fast-response voicing trigger mechanism is still open to debate, but the dimension of the tension control of the vocal fold seems to be another important correlate of laryngeal articulatory adjustment.

LARYNGEAL MUSCLE ACTIONS IN THE SUPRASEGMENTAL (PROSODIC) CONTROL OF SPEECH

EMG studies of the laryngeal muscles during speech in a variety of languages have shown that these muscles are primarily responsible for pitch (F_0) control, no matter what type of pitch change is involved (Ohala, 1978).

The principal mechanism for pitch change is an increase or decrease in the longitudinal tension of the vocal fold, and the function of the CT is certainly related to this process. However, the mechanism of pitch lowering is not as straightforward as that of pitch elevation. As for the contribution of the external laryngeal muscles (the so-called strap muscle group) to pitch lowering, their activities often appear to be a result, rather than the cause, of change in conditions, lacking a lead in time relative to the physical effects of pitch change.

Figure 18-6 shows examples of the EMG curves of the LCA, CT, and sternohyoid (SH) for single tokens of isolated, two-mora Japanese words with four contrasting accent patterns from the Kinki dialect (Sugito and Hirose, 1978).

It is obvious that CT activation is related to pitch rise with some lead in time. As for pitch lowering, the

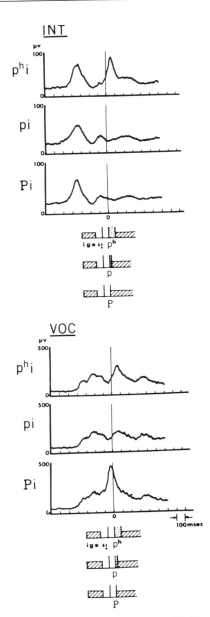

Figure 18-4. *Averaged EMG curves of INT and VOC for the three bilabial stops of Korean in word-initial position. The zero on the abscissa marks the line-up point for the averaging and corresponds to the stop release.*

decrease in CT activity and increase in SH appear to correlate
with the F_0 contour, particularly in
accent types A and B. However,
there is an apparent time delay between the onset of the decline in
CT activity and that of the elevation
of SH activity in type A. Thus, SH
seems to play a role in assisting or
enhancing a sharp descent of F_0,
as shown in these cases, although
it is not likely that the SH acts as
the primary pitch lowering muscle.

It is interesting to note that there
is SH activation before the voice
onset in the so-called low-start
types B and C. The increase in SH
activity before the voice onset has
been found in other cases as well
and has been interpreted as an indication of the contribution of the
SH to preparing the larynx for the
speech mode in certain specific
cases (Sawashima and Hirose,
1983). This possibility needs further investigation.

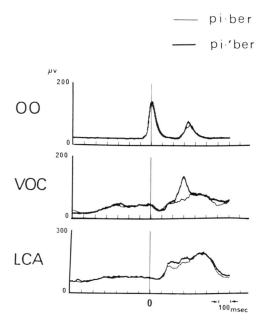

Figure 18-5. *Averaged EMG curves of the orbicularis oris (OO), VOC, and LCA for Danish test words with and without "stød."*

CONCLUDING REMARKS

In this paper, several topics related to laryngeal control in speech
articulation are presented. It
should be emphasized that the
human larynx is not simply an
organ of phonation, but serves as
an important organ for speech.
The adjustment of the laryngeal
muscles in voiceless consonant
production is particularly unique in
that the laryngeal abductor, the
PCA, is activated even during the
phase of expiration.

It is hoped that further research
will clarify the role of the human
larynx in both phonation and
articulation.

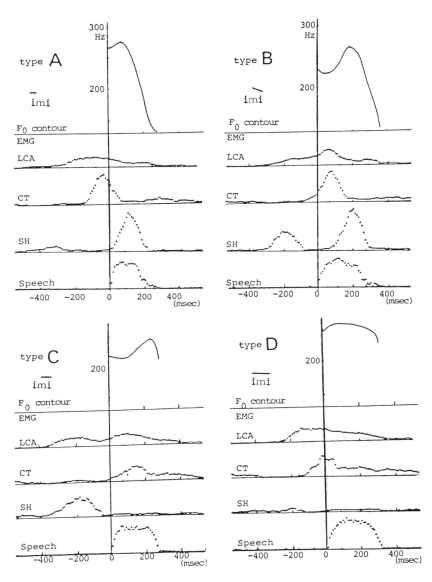

Figure 18-6. *Smoothed and integrated EMG curves of the LCA, CT, and SH, and pitch contours for single tokens of two-mora Japanese words having four different accent patterns from the Kinki dialect. The vertical bar indicates the onset of voicing.*

REFERENCES

Benguerel, A-P., Hirose, H., Sawashima, M., and Ushijima, T. (1978). Laryngeal control in French stop production: A fiberoptic, acoustic and electromyographic study. *Folia Phoniat, 30,* 175–198.

Dixit, R.P. (1975). *Neuromuscular aspects of laryngeal control: With special reference to Hindi.* Unpublished doctoral dissertation, University of Texas at Austin.

Fischer-Jorgensen, E., and Hirose, H. (1974). A preliminary electromyographic study of labial and laryngeal muscles in Danish stop consonant production. *Haskins Laboratories Status Report on Speech Research, SR-39/40,* 231–254.

Hirano, M. (1975). Phonosurgery. Basic and clinical investigations. *Otologia Fukuoka, 21,* (Suppl. 1), 239–442.

Hirose, H. (1961). Afferent impulses in the recurrent laryngeal nerve in the cat. *Laryngoscope, 71,* 1196–1206.

Hirose, H. (1976). Posterior cricoarytenoid as a speech muscle. *Ann Otol Rhinol Laryngol, 75,* 334–343.

Hirose, H. (1977). Laryngeal adjustments in consonant production. *Phonetica, 34,* 289–294.

Hirose, H., and Gay, T. (1972). The activity of the intrinsic laryngeal muscles in voicing control; Electromyographic study. *Phonetica, 25,* 140–164.

Hirose, H., Lee, C.Y., and Ushijima, T. (1974). Laryngeal control in Korean stop production. *J Phonetics, 2,* 145–152.

Hirose, H., Lisker, L., and Abramson, A. (1972). Physiological aspects of certain laryngeal features in stop production. *Haskins Laboratories Status Report on Speech Research, SR-31/32,* 183–191.

Hirose, H., and Sawashima, M. (1981). Functions of the laryngeal muscles in speech. In K N. Stevens, and M. Hirano, (Eds.), *Vocal Fold Physiology* (pp. 137–154). Tokyo: University of Tokyo Press.

Hirose, H., Sawashima, M., and Yoshioka, H. (1983). Laryngeal adjustment for initiation of utterance: A simultaneous EMG and fiberoptic study. In D.M. Bless and J.H. Abbs (Eds.), *Vocal Fold Physiology* (pp. 253–263). San Diego: College-Hill Press.

Hirose, H., and Ushijima, T. (1978). Laryngeal control for voicing distinction in Japanese consonant production. *Phonetica, 35,* 1–10.

Hirose, H., Yoshioka, H., and Niimi, S. (1979). A cross language study of laryngeal adjustment in consonant production. In H. Hollien and P. Hollien (Eds.), *Amsterdam studies in the theory and history of linguistic science IV. Current issues in linguistic theory Vol. 9. Current issues in the phonetic sciences* (pp. 165–179). Amsterdam: John-Benjamin, B.V.

Kagaya, R., and Hirose, H. (1975). Fiberoptic, electromyographic and acoustic analysis of Hindi stop consonants. *Ann Bull RILP, 9,* 27–46.

Ohala, J.J. (1967). The production of tone. Report of phonology lab. *University of California at Berkeley, 2,* 63–117.

Sawashima, M., and Hirose, H. (1983). Laryngeal gestures in speech production. In P. F. MacNeilage (Ed.), *The production of speech* (pp. 11–38). New York: Springer-Verlag.

Sugito, M., and Hirose, H. (1978). An electromyographic study of Kinki accent. *Ann Bull RILP, 12,* 35–52.

Yoshioka, H., Lofqvist, A., and Hirose, H. (1981). Laryngeal adjustments in the production of consonant clusters and geminates in American English. *Jour Acoust Soc Amer, 70,* 1615–1623.

CHAPTER 19

The Laryngeal Muscles in Singing

Minoru HIRANO

Human beings, especially singers, can produce great varieties of vibratory patterns and subsequent tonal variations with the use of only one sound generator, a pair of vocal folds. This is in contrast to many musical instruments. A piano, violin, or guitar, for instance, requires multiple sound generators in order to produce variations in tone. In other words, the human vocal folds can become vibrators that have different mechanical properties and subsequent vibratory characteristics.

This remarkable versatility in sound production is possible because of two properties of the human vocal folds: (1) they are subject to fine grained and delicate muscular control, and (2) their structure is ideally suited for the

task, because of being layered and physically pliable (Hirano, 1975; 1981a; 1981c).

We have investigated the function of the laryngeal muscles, related directly or indirectly to singing, over the past two decades (Hirano, Ohala, and Vennard, 1969; Hirano, 1970a, 1970b; Hirano, Vennard, and Ohala, 1970; Hirano, 1971; Hirano, Miyahara, Miyagi, 1971; Hirano, 1981b; 1982). This paper describes summaries of the results of our series of works. There is no doubt that varying singing techniques are associated with different muscular controls. Delicate differences in muscular control can cause subtle variations of voice quality. Each singer has his or her own individuality in this regard. This paper cannot go into such subtleties, but rather focuses on functions of the laryngeal muscles that are common to the subjects we have investigated.

BASIC FUNCTION OF LARYNGEAL MUSCLES

The basic function of each intrinsic laryngeal muscle, as investigated with excised canine larynges, will be described in this section. Although there are some differences in structure between human and canine larynges (Hirano, 1975; 1981a), the basic gross function of the major laryngeal muscles, that is, the cricothyroid (CT), thyroarytenoid or vocalis (VOC), lateral cricoarytenoid (LCA), interarytenoid (IA), and posterior cricoarytenoid (PCA) muscles, is qualitatively the same for the two species (Takase, 1964).

Figures 19-1 and 19-2A,B,C,D show pictures of canine larynges taken when each of the laryngeal muscles of freshly excised larynges was electrically stimulated. Figure 19-3A,B,C,D shows histological pictures of a frontal section at the middle of the membranous vocal fold. The histological specimens were obtained by fixing the larynx in −30°C alcohol during electrical stimulation.

CT Activation

The vocal fold is stretched, elongated, thinned, and slightly adducted to the paramedian position. The level of the vocal fold within the larynx is lowered. The edge of the vocal fold becomes sharp. The cross sectional area of the mucosa and that of the muscle are decreased. Both mucosa

and muscle are supposed to be passively stiffened.

VOC Activation

The vocal fold is adducted, especially at the membranous portion. It is also shortened and thickened. The level of the vocal fold within the larynx is lowered. The edge of the vocal fold is rounded. The cross sectional area of the mucosa and that of the muscle are increased. The mucosa appears to be slackened, whereas the muscle is stiffened by its own contraction.

LCA Activation

The tip of the vocal process is adducted and lowered, resulting in adduction and lowering of the entire vocal fold. The vocal fold is elongated and thinned. The edge of the vocal fold becomes sharp. The cross sectional area of the mucosa and that of the muscle are reduced. Both mucosa and muscle appear to be passively stiffened.

IA Activation

The arytenoid region is adducted, closing the posterior part of the larynx. The membranous vocal fold is adducted to some extent. The vocal fold is slightly shortened, thickened, and slackened.

PCA Activation

The tip of the vocal process is abducted and elevated, resulting in abduction and elevation of the entire vocal fold. The vocal fold is markedly elongated and becomes

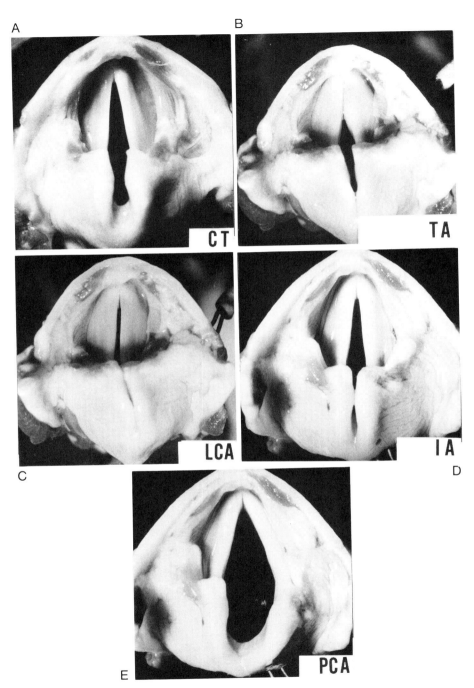

Figure 19-1. *Position and shape of canine vocal fold during electrical stimulation of each laryngeal muscle. View from above. A: CT, B: TA, C: LCA, D: IA, E: PCA stimulated (Hirano, 1975).*

thin. The edge of the vocal fold is rounded. The cross sectional area of the mucosa and that of the muscle are decreased. Both mucosa and muscle are supposed to be passively stiffened.

Table 19-1 summarizes functions of the five major laryngeal muscles.

CONTROL OF VOCAL REGISTER

There are three major vocal registers: falsetto or light, modal or heavy, and vocal fry. Falsetto is characterized by the absence of complete glottal closure. The modal register is accompanied by complete glottal closure for each vibratory cycle, and it is traditionally subdivided into head, mid, and chest registers. Vocal fry is characterized by an extremely long closed phase relative to one vibratory cycle. Occasionally, it has two open phases during one vibratory cycle. Our investigations have focused primarily on the falsetto and modal registers. Investigations on vocal fry were rather limited.

Comparison of Muscular Activity among Different Registers at the Same Pitch

Muscular activity was compared among sustained tones phonated in different registers, but at the same pitch, by means of EMG (Hirano and Ohala, 1969). Four singers served as the subjects for this study. Table 19-2 summarizes the results of these comparisons.

As is apparent from Table 19-2, the heavier the register, the great-

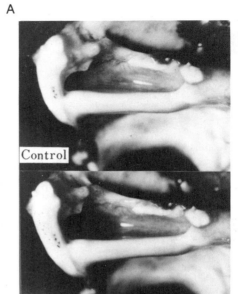

A

B

Figure 19-2. *Position and shape of canine vocal fold during electrical stimulation of each laryngeal muscle. View from inside. A: CT, B: TA, C: LCA, D: PCA (Hirano, 1975).*

(continued on page 213)

er the VOC activity in all four subjects. The only exception was observed at pitch G_3 of subject W.V., in which the VOC activity was approximately the same for the head and chest registers. LCA tended also to be more active for the heavier register, but not as consistently as VOC. In addition, the difference in LCA activity was not as marked as that in VOC activity. The activity of IA, which was investigated in only one subject, was slightly greater for the heavier register. The activity of CT did not show any consistent relationship to changes in vocal register.

Figure 19-4 illustrates muscle activity and acoustic recordings from one subject.

Muscular Activity Pattern in Response to Register Shift

The muscular activity pattern was investigated when the vocal register was shifted during singing. Scales, arpeggios, vocalises, and parts of songs were employed as the phonation samples. Five singers served as the subjects for these tasks. Table 19-3 summarizes the results of this study.

As shown, VOC always presented a marked change in activity in response to register shifts. Register shifts from heavy to light were accompanied by a decrease in VOC activity, whereas shifts to heavier registers were associated with VOC increases. The direction of the changes in the LCA, CT, and IA activity were the same as in the case of the VOC. However, in the LCA, changes in activity accompanied by register shifts were observed less consistently, and changes in CT activity were even

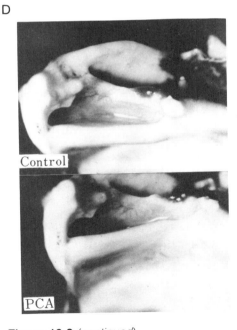

Figure 19-2 (*continued*).

less consistent. IA, investigated in one subject, also showed changes in activities associated with register shifts.

Figures 19-5, 19-6, 19-7 and 19-8 show examples of raw EMG recordings demonstrating changes in muscular activity associated with register shifts.

Muscular Activity for Vocal Fry

Our electromyographic study of vocal fry has been very limited. VOC and IA were investigated in only one subject, an untrained male.

Figure 19-9 shows VOC activity when the subject produced vocal fry followed by an ascending scale in the modal voice. VOC activity for the vocal fry was about the same as that for the low pitched modal voice, but smaller than that for the high pitched modal voice. The airflow was much smaller for the vocal fry than for the modal voice.

Figure 19-10 shows IA activity of the same subject when he produced vocal fry followed by a low modal voice at pitch C_3. IA activity was larger for the modal voice than for the vocal fry.

Figure 19-11 compares the view of the larynx of the same subject between a modal voice at a low pitch and a vocal fry. In the modal voice, the vocal folds were short and their edges were blurred because of vibrations. The edges appeared slackened and pliable. In the vocal fry, the vocal folds were shorter, the glottis was closed more tightly, and the ventricular folds were adducted to a greater extent than in the modal voice. However, the arytenoids were

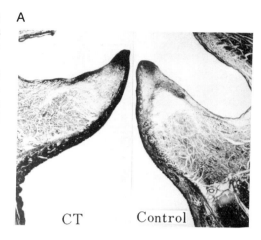

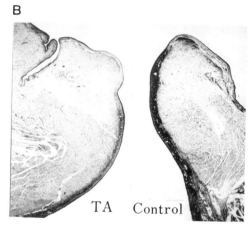

Figure 19-3. *Histological presentation of structural changes in canine vocal fold caused by electrical stimulation of each laryngeal muscle. A: CT, B: TA, C: LCA, D: PCA (Hirano, 1975).*

(continued on page 215)

approximated to a lesser extent than in the modal voice.

The lesser extent of the arytenoid approximation in vocal fry can be attributed to less IA activity. The tighter closure of the glottis for vocal fry cannot be accounted for by VOC activity because VOC did not present greater activity in vocal fry. We presume that there should be a marked lateral compression of the vocal folds in vocal fry, probably brought about by the outer portion of TA and the thyropharyngeal muscle.

Adjustments of the Layer Structured Vocal Fold for Different Registers

The vocal fold, the vibrator for sound production, has a layered structure (Hirano, 1975; 1981a). On the basis of the results of EMG studies described so far, adjustments of the layer structure of the vocal fold for different registers will be discussed in this section (Figure 19-12).

In vocal fry, VOC activity is minimum. CT activity is presumably minimum, too, because the vocal folds are very short. Therefore, all the layers are supposed to be slackened and pliant. There is, however, a large lateral compression, resulting in a large glottal resistance. When the vocal folds adjusted in this way are set into motion, vibrations of a long closed phase result.

In the modal voice, VOC activity is dominant over CT activity. As the fundamental frequency (F_0) increases, both VOC and CT activities increase. However, VOC remains dominant. Therefore, the body is stiffer than the cover and

C

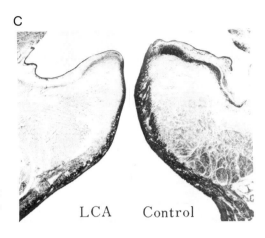

LCA   Control

D

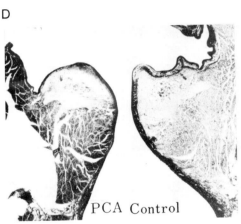

PCA Control

Figure 19-3 (*continued*).

TABLE 19-1.
Functions of the Five Major Laryngeal Muscles in Vocal Fold Adjustment.

	CT	VOC	LCA	IA	PCA
Position	Paramed	*Adduct*	*Adduct*	*Adduct*	*Abduct*
Level	Lower	Lower	*Lower*	0	*Elevate*
Length	*Elongate*	*Shorten*	Elongate	(Shorten)	*Elongate*
Thickness	*Thin*	*Thicken*	Thin	(Thicken)	Thin
Edge	*Sharpen*	*Round*	Sharpen	0	Round
Muscle (Body)	*Stiffen*	*Stiffen*	Stiffen	(Slacken)	Stiffen
Mucosa (Cover and transition)	*Stiffen*	*Slacken*	Stiffen	(Slacken)	Stiffen

0: No effect, ( ): Slightly, In italics: Markedly
Hirano, 1981c.

TABLE 19-2.
Degree of Muscular Activity as Shown in Rank Order. The Activity of Each Muscle is Compared among Different Registers at the Same Fundamental Frequency.

Subject	Fundamental pitch	Register	CT	LCA	VOC	IA
J. R. (Soprano)	G_4	Head	2	3	3	
		Mid	3	2	2	
		Chest	1	1	1	
M. M. (Tenor)	C_4	Falsetto	2	3	3	
		Head	2	2	2	
		Chest	2	1	1	
T. M. (Tenor)	C_4	Falsetto	3	3	3	
		Mid	1	1.5	2	
		Chest	2	1.5	1	
W. V. (Bass)	G_3	Falsetto	3	3	3	
		Head	1.5	2	1.5	
		Chest	1.5	1	1.5	
	C_4	Falsetto	2.5	2.5	3	3
		Head	1	1	2	2
		Chest	2.5	2.5	1	1

Hirano, 1975.

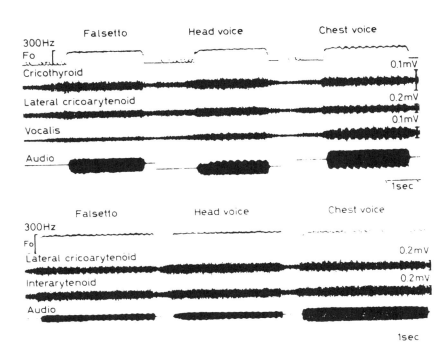

Figure 19-4. Activity of CT, LCA, VOC, and IA in different vocal registers at the same fundamental frequency (C₄) (Hirano et al., 1970).

TABLE 19-3.
Changes in Muscular Activity in Response to Register Shift during Singing.

Subject	CT	LCA	VOC	IA
L. C. (Soprano)	(+) or −	+ or −	+	
J. R. (Soprano)	(+) or −	+		
M. M. (Tenor)	(+) or −	+ or −	+	
T. M. (Tenor)	(+) or −	+ or −	+	
W. V. (Bass)	(+) or −	+ or −	+	+

+ : Change found
( ): Not frequent
− : Change not found
Hirano, 1975.

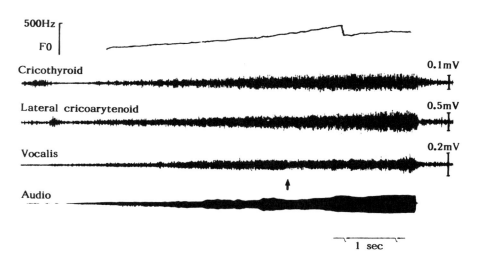

Figure 19-5. *Activity of CT, LCA, and VOC during singing of 3-octave scale ascending (F_2-F_5). Arrow indicates register transition from chest to head associated with marked decrease in VOC activity (Hirano et al., 1970).*

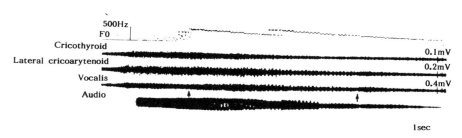

Figure 19-6. *Activity of CT, LCA, and VOC during singing of 3-octave scale descending (E^b_6–E^b_3). Arrows indicate register transitions from falsetto to head (left arrow) and from mid to chest (right arrow), both associated with increased VOC activity (Hirano et al., 1970).*

transition. In the cover and transition, the elastic fibers in the vocal ligament oppose the stretching force brought about by the CT. The collagenous fibers are not fully stretched, and, therefore, more or less slackened and pliable. This vocal fold adjustment results in a vibratory pattern which consists of an opening phase, closing phase, and closed phase and is associated with the mucosal wave.

The modal voice can be subclassified into head voice, mid voice, and chest voice. These differences are supposed to depend chiefly on the balance between VOC activity and CT activity. For example, Figure 19-4 shows that VOC activity is greater for a chest voice than for a head voice at the same pitch level, whereas CT activity is higher for the head voice than for the chest. General-

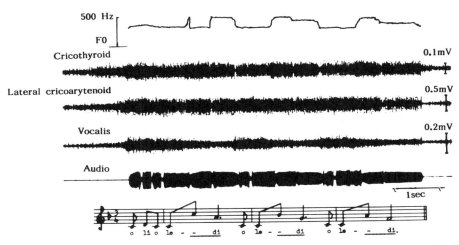

Figure 19-7. *Activity of CT, LCA, and VOC during yodeling. Underlined parts were yodeled in falsetto. VOC activity is markedly decreased for yodeling. CT activity is slightly increased during yodeling in order to raise F_0. LCA does not present marked activity change. Activity increase for high F_0 and decrease for falsetto should be balanced (Hirano et al., 1970).*

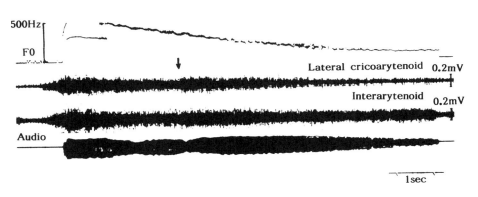

Figure 19-8. *Activity of LCA and IA during singing of 3-octave scale descending (D_5–D_2). Arrow indicates register transition from falsetto to head associated with activity increase of LCA and IA (Hirano et al., 1970).*

ly speaking, as CT activity becomes greater relative to VOC activity, the voice changes from chest to mid, and mid to head.

Of course, the other intrinsic and extrinsic laryngeal muscles also affect the mechanical properties of each layer of the vocal folds (Hirano 1975; 1981a). Contribution of the supraglottic and subglottic tubes to the vocal register should not be overlooked. However, the principal register agents appear to be VOC and CT.

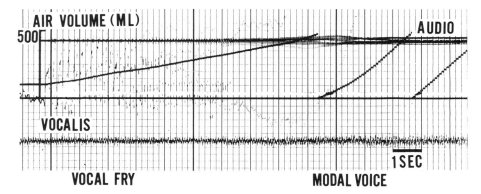

Figure 19-9. *VOC activity during production of vocal fry followed by ascending scale (Hirano, 1982).*

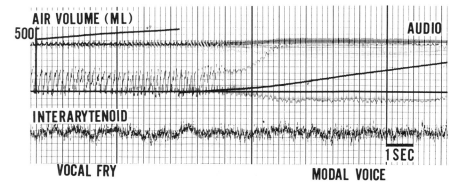

Figure 19-10. *IA activity during production of vocal fry followed by low modal voice (Hirano, 1982).*

In falsetto, VOC contracts weakly or completely relaxes. CT is active to a significant degree. Therefore, all the layers of the vocal folds are stretched. In this condition, the collagenous fibers in the vocal ligament should be the stiffest in all the layers. Furthermore, because CT can abduct the vocal fold when it is in the median position, the glottis is slightly open. This vocal fold adjustment produces a vibratory pattern which has no closed phase.

CONTROL OF FUNDAMENTAL FREQUENCY (F_0) OF VOICE

The function of the laryngeal muscles in regulating F_0 depended on the vocal register.

F_0 Regulation in Modal Register

The relationships between muscular activities and F_0 were investigated in five singers and four untrained subjects. The results are summarized in Table 19-4. In the modal register, the activity of CT, LCA, and VOC were always positively related to F_0 (as shown in Figures 19-5, 19-6, 19-8 and 19-13). IA presented greater activity at the higher F_0. There were, however, no gradual changes in IA activity closely related to F_0 (as shown in Figure 19-8). PCA was investigated in only one subject. It was usually inactive during phonation, with the exception of high tones in the modal register (Figure 19-13). This activity of PCA is presumably required in order to brace the arytenoid cartilage against the strong anterior pull of the CT.

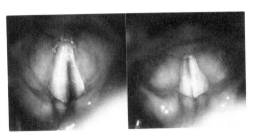

Figure 19-11. Views of larynx during phonation in modal voice at low pitch (left) and in vocal fry (right) (Hirano, 1982).

F_0 Regulation in Falsetto

F_0 regulation in falsetto was investigated in five singers. Table 19-5 summarizes the results. In contrast to the case in modal register, the activity of CT, LCA, and VOC was not always positively related to F_0 in falsetto. However, in a given singing sample, it was rare that none of these three muscles showed activities positively related to F_0. It is worth noting that CT, which plays the most important role in F_0 control in the modal register, did not always contribute in falsetto. The IA activity was greater at the higher F_0, but it was not closely related to F_0.

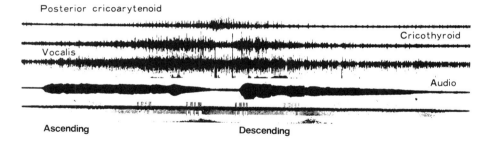

Posterior cricoarytenoid

Cricothyroid

Vocalis

Audio

Ascending   Descending

Figure 19-12. *Schematic presentation of variation of layer structure of vocal folds for different registers (Hirano, 1982).*

TABLE 19-4.
Relation of Muscular Activity to Fundamental Frequency in the Modal Register.

	Subject	CT	LCA	VOC	IA	PCA
	L. C. (Soprano)	+	+	+		
	J. R. (Soprano)	+	+			
Professional singer	M. M. (Tenor)	+	+	+		
	T. M. (Tenor)	+	+	+		
	W. V. (Bass)	+	+	+	+ or 0	
	J. O.	+	+	+	+ or 0	
Untrained	D. B.	+	+			
	J. A.	+	+			
	H. H.	+	+	+	+ or 0	+ or 0

+: Positively related, 0: Not related.
Hirano, 1975.

CONTROL OF VOCAL INTENSITY

Muscular activity was investigated when the vocal intensity was changed gradually, as in crescendo, decrescendo, and swelltone at the same F_0 level. In some subjects, comparisons were attempted among separate tones produced at different intensities, but at the same F_0 and in the same register. There were great inter- and intrasubject variations in the EMG data in this latter case. The expiratory effort appeared to vary

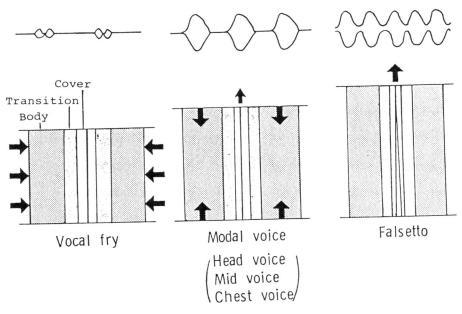

Figure 19-13. *Activity of PCA, CT, and VOC during singing of ascending and descending scales in modal register (Hirano, 1975).*

more substantially and in less systematic ways than in the case of gradual intensity changes.

Intensity Regulation in Modal Register

The results of the regulation of intensity in the modal register are shown in Table 19-6. The muscle that exhibited the greatest variation in activity with changes in intensity was VOC. Especially in singers, the activity of VOC changed markedly in proportion to the vocal intensity irrespective of the F_0 level. In untrained subjects, a similar kind of change was observed for low F_0. However, the degree of change in activity was not so great as in the case of singers. For high F_0, VOC did not contribute to intensity regulation in untrained subjects. These findings suggest that a good command of VOC control is one of the most important factors in the proficiency of voice technique.

LCA and IA activity increased with the vocal intensity, but less consistently than VOC. CT activity was often inversely related to the vocal intensity. The expiratory air pressure and glottal resistance, changes of which accompany vocal intensity increases, can also cause a rise in F_0. As such, CT activity may have to be proportionally reduced to maintain a constant F_0 level. PCA was activated only at high F_0 and had activity level changes similar to CT.

TABLE 19-5.
Relation of Muscular Activity to Fundamental Frequency in the Falsetto Register.

Subject	CT	LCA	VOC	IA
L. C. (Soprano)	+ or 0	+	+ or 0	
J. R. (Soprano)	+ or 0	+		
M. M. (Tenor)	+ or 0	+ or 0	+ or 0	
T. M. (Tenor)	+	+	0	
W. V. (Bass)	+ or 0	+	+	+ or 0

+: Positively related. 0: Not related.
Hirano, 1975.

TABLE 19-6.
Relation of Muscular Activity to Intensity of Voice in the Modal Register.

Subject		Fundamental pitch	CT	LCA	VOC	IA	PCA
	L. C. (Soprano)	D_4	−	0	+		
		G_4	−	− ~ +	+		
		D_5	−	− ~ +	+		
	J. R. (Soprano)	C_4	− or 0				
		G_4	−	+ or 0			
		C_5	−	−			
Professional singer	M. M. (Tenor)	C_4	−	+	+		
		G_4	− ~ +	+			
	T. M. (Tenor)	F_3	−	−	+		
		F_4	−	−	+		
		A_4	−	−	+		
	W. V. (Bass)	C_3	0	+	+	−	
		G_3	0	+	+	+	
		C_4	−	− or 0	+	0	
Untrained	J. O.	C_3			+	+	
		G_3			+ or 0	+	
		C_4			0	+	
	H. H.	low	0		+		0
		high	−		0		−

+: Positively related, 0: Not related, −: Negatively related, − ~ +: Negatively related at a lesser intensity, and positively related at a greater intensity.
Hirano, 1975.

Intensity Regulation in Falsetto

Table 19-7 summarizes the results for intensity regulation in falsetto. In falsetto, none of the muscles showed any evidence of a significant contribution to intensity control. This indicates that the vocal intensity is regulated almost exclusively by the expiratory air pressure. As in the modal register, CT activity varied inversely with the vocal intensity, probably to maintain F_0 at a constant level, as mentioned earlier.

CONTROL OF VOCAL ONSET

Muscular activities of three singers were investigated for four types of vocal onsets: soft, hard, breathy, and imaginary H onset. The subjects produced the vowel /a/ at their habitual F_0 and intensity following signals given with a baton. The timing of the prephonatory inspiration and the voice onset was controlled in this way. Each onset was repeated ten times. Figure 19-14A,B,C,D depicts EMG recordings for the four onset types.

Table 19-8 shows duration of the prephonatory muscular activity in each singer. As shown, there were marked intra- and intersubject variations in the values obtained. No systematic differences in the duration of the prephonatory activity were found among different onset types or among the muscles.

Table 19-9 compares the amplitude of muscular activities between, before, and during phonation as well as among different voice onset types. The adductor muscles, that is, the LCA and VOC, presented unique activity patterns

TABLE 19-7.
Relation of Muscular Activity to Intensity of Voice in the Falsetto Register.

	Subject	Fundamental pitch	CT	LCA	VOC	IA
Professional singer	L. C. (Soprano)	E_6	−	0	0	
	J. R. (Soprano)	C_6	− or 0	+		
	M. M. (Tenor)	G_4 C_5	− −	0 0	+ or 0 0	
	T. M. (Tenor)	F_4	−	−	0	
	W. V. (Bass)	C_4 G_4	− −	− −	0 −	−
Untrained	J. O.	A_4				0

+: Positively related, 0: Not related, −: Negatively related.
Hirano, 1975.

for the hard onset. Their prephonatory activity was greater than the activity during phonation for the hard onset. Their prephonatory activity was also greater for the hard onset than for the other onset types.

In the soft and imaginary H onset, the activity of CT, LCA, and VOC increased gradually and reached the maximum level around the vocal onset. No difference in activity pattern was found between these two onset types. However, the voice onset was clearer in the imaginary H onset than in the soft onset. In the hard onset, the activity of LCA and VOC increased rapidly to reach a markedly high level. Their activity decreased abruptly immediately before the voice onset and then increased again to the level during phonation. CT showed a gradual increase in activity even for the hard onset. In the breathy onset, the activity of CT, LCA, and VOC increased gradually to reach the phonation level. Occasionally, the activity of LCA and VOC showed a temporary weakening during the gradual increase.

COMMENTS

Vocal control during singing is achieved by coordinated functions of the respiratory, laryngeal, and articulatory muscles. The laryngeal muscles directly regulate the mechanical characteristics of the vocal fold. Each laryngeal muscle participates in regulating not only one vocal parameter, but two or more parameters.

CT is basically a F_0 agent. It increases F_0 by tensing the vocal fold. CT also opposes VOC with respect to the tension of the vocal

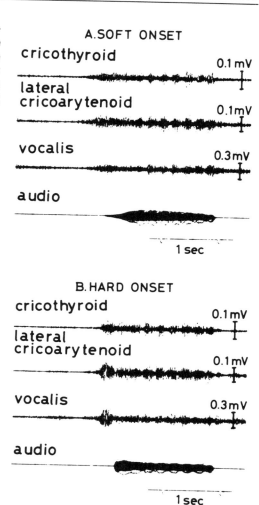

Figure 19-14. *Activity of CT, LCA, and VOC for different voice onset types.*

(continued on page 227)

fold mucosa. In this way, CT also participates greatly in regulating vocal register. An increase in F_0 tends to be associated with a register shift from heavy to light, whereas a decrease in F_0 is likely to be associated with a register change from light to heavy.

VOC loosens and thickens the vocal fold mucosa. Loose and thick mucosa is essential for heavy register. VOC also increases the glottal resistance. An increase in glottal resistance is one of the most important factors contributing to an increase in vocal intensity. In these ways, VOC plays important roles in regulating the vocal register and intensity.

LCA participates in control of vocal register, F_0, and vocal intensity. It is not a leading actor, but an important supporting actor.

IA does not affect the mechanical characteristics of the vibrator as greatly as the previous three muscles do. Its main role is to close the glottis. It seems, however, that IA supports other muscles in controlling vocal register, F_0, and vocal intensity.

VOC, LCA, and IA are referred to as the adductors of the vocal fold. Their roles in singing are not simply adduction of the vocal fold; each of the adductors, especially VOC and LCA, has a different and important role in addition to adduction.

PCA is the abductor of the vocal fold and basically participates in inspiration. Under a special condition, however, it seems to participate in controlling the singing voice.

Table 19-10 summarizes the contributions of the laryngeal muscles in the regulation of important parameters of the singing voice.

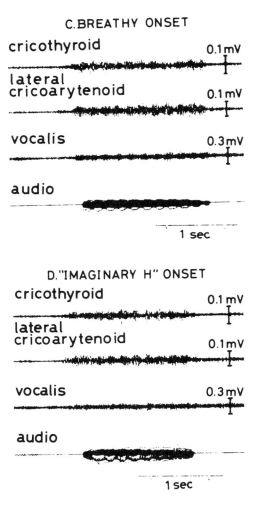

Figure 19-14 (*continued*).

TABLE 19-8.

Duration of Prephonatory Muscular Activity for Different Voice Onset Types. Mean Value and Range (in Parentheses) for Ten Utterances.

Subject	Onset	CT	LCA	VOC
L. C. Soprano	Soft	1050 (720-1240)	1170 (840-1720)	890 (640-1120)
	Hard	1020 (720-1360)	1130 (720-1600)	810 (560-1000)
	Breathy	1210 (720-1600)	1220 (800-1680)	1080 (680-1360)
	Imaginary H	1010 (720-1320)	1010 (720-1280)	850 (720-1040)
J. R. Soprano	Soft	990 (560-1360)	1030 (800-1320)	
	Hard	890 (640-1120)	740 (600-1040)	
	Breathy	860 (480-1200)	320 (160- 640)	
	Imaginary H	920 (720-1600)	860 (440-1520)	
W. V. Bass	Soft	390 (345- 425)	585 (505- 690)	470 (345- 660)
	Hard	385 (290- 530)	450 (370- 530)	410 (290- 500)
	Breathy	460 (330- 635)	520 (370- 610)	425 (320- 530)
	Imaginary H	370 (320- 450)	480 (400- 530)	430 (345- 660)

Hirano, 1971.

TABLE 19-9.
Maximum Amplitude of Muscular Activity before and during Phonation for Different Voice Onset Types. Mean Value and Range (in Parentheses) for Ten Utterances.

Subj.	Onset	CT		LCA		VOC	
		Before	During	Before	During	Before	During
L. C. Sopr.	Soft	80 (60-90)	85 (75-90)	170 (140-230)	150 (110-230)	220 (180-270)	220 (180-270)
	Hard	90 (75-100)	70 (60-90)	230 (180-250)	170 (140-200)	460 (400-540)	350 (270-400)
	Breathy	80 (60-90)	80 (60-90)	170 (140-200)	150 (110-180)	260 (220-270)	260 (220-270)
	Imagin. H	75 (60-90)	75 (60-90)	140 (110-160)	140 (110-160)	220 (180-270)	230 (220-270)
J. R. Sopr.	Soft	105 (100-110)	105 (100-110)	240 (190-290)	240 (220-290)		
	Hard	110 (100-130)	110 (100-130)	250 (200-290)	200 (160-260)		
	Breathy	100 (100-110)	105 (100-110)	200 (190-220)	250 (220-290)		
	Imagin. H	110 (100-160)	105 (100-155)	210 (190-220)	215 (190-260)		
W. V. Bass	Soft	90 (50-130)	115 (100-135)	85 (70-105)	155 (85-110)	100 (100-210)	175 (150-200)
	Hard	130 (100-150)	135 (115-170)	160 (140-175)	90 (80-105)	370 (335-430)	165 (140-190)
	Breathy	90 (60-120)	135 (115-155)	75 (60-90)	90 (75-90)	125 (100-155)	155 (130-190)
	Imagin. H	85 (70-95)	120 (110-140)	70 (65-80)	90 (75-105)	120 (100-140)	145 (115-165)

Subj.: Subject, Sopr.: Soprano, Imagin.: Imaginary
Hirano, 1971.

TABLE 19-10.

Contribution of the Laryngeal Muscles to Regulation of Vocal Register, Fundamental Frequency (FO) and Vocal Intensity

	Register	FO		Intensity
CT	#	Light	+	−
		Heavy	#	−
VOC	#	Light	±	−
		Heavy	+	#
LCA	+	Light	±	−
		Heavy	+	±
IA	+	Light	±	−
		Heavy	±	±
PCA	−	Light	−	−
		Heavy	±	−
Respiratory muscles*	−	−		#

#: Marked contribution, +: Some contribution, ±: Occasional contribution, −: Little or no contribution, *: Based on separate aerodynamic studies.

REFERENCES

Hirano, M. (1970a). Regulatory mechanism of voice in singing. *J. Logoped Phoniat. Jpn. 11*, 1–11.

Hirano, M. (1970b). *Regulatory mechanism of voice in singing.* [16mm Film]. Kurume: Karume University.

Hirano, M. (1971). Laryngeal adjustment for different vocal onsets. *J Otolaryngol Jpn 74*, 1572–1579.

Hirano, M. (1975). Phonosurgery. Basic and clinical investigations. *Otologia Fukuoka, 21*, 239–440.

Hirano, M. (1981a). Structure of the vocal fold in normal and disease states. Anatomical and physical studies. *ASHA Report, 11*, 11–30.

Hirano, M. (1981b). The function of the intrinsic laryngeal muscles in singing. In K.N. Stevens and M. Hirano (Eds.), *Vocal fold physiology* (pp. 155–170). Tokyo: University of Tokyo Press.

Hirano, M. (1981c). *Clinical examination of voice.* New York: Springer-Verlag.

Hirano, M. (1982). The role of the layer structure of the vocal fold in register control. In P. Hurme (Ed.), *Vox humana* (pp. 50–62). Jyvaeskylae: University of Jyvaeskylae.

Hirano, M., Miyahara, T., Miyagi, T. (1971). Vocal regulation in singing. An experimental study in a professional singer. *J Otolaryngol Jpn 74*, 1189–1201.

Hirano, M., and Ohala, J. (1969). Use of hooked-wire electrodes for electromyography of the intrinsic laryngeal muscles. *J. Speech Hearing Res. 12*, 362–372.

Hirano, M., Ohala, J., and Vennard, W. (1969). The function of laryngeal muscles in regulating fundamental frequency and intensity of phonation. *J. Speech Hearing Res. 12*, 616–628.

Hirano, M., Vennard, W., and Ohala, J. (1970). Regulation of register, pitch and intensity of voice. An electromyographic investigation of intrinsic laryngeal muscles. *Folia Phoniat. 22*, 1–20.

Takase, S. (1964). Studies on the intrinsic laryngeal muscles of mammals. Comparative anatomy and physiology. *Otologia Fukuoka 10*, (Suppl. 1), 18–58.

PART 5

Pathology

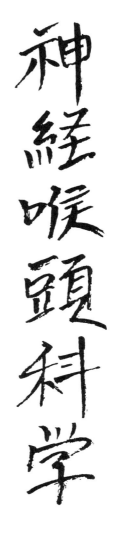

CHAPTER 20

Electromyography for Laryngeal Paralysis

Minoru HIRANO,
Isao NOZOE,
Takemoto SHIN
and Tadatsugu MAEYAMA

Electromyography (EMG) is a useful procedure for making diagnostic and prognostic decisions in cases of neuromuscular diseases. Basically, EMG can be applied to cases of laryngeal paralysis in the same way as it can to paralysis of the skeletal muscles. EMG is also useful in discussing the pathophysiology of laryngeal paralysis.

This paper is a modified version of our paper that was originally written in Japanese (Hirano, Nozoe, Shin, and Maeyama, 1974). It focuses primarily on the timing of components of EMG patterns, the differences in vulnerability and recovery among the muscles innervated by the recurrent laryngeal nerve (RLN), the relationship between the location of the paretic vocal fold and EMG findings, the relationship between the etiology of the paralysis and EMG patterns, and the prognostic uses of EMG.

SUBJECTS AND METHODS

During the period 1963 to 1970, 130 EMG sessions were conducted with 114 cases of unilateral laryngeal paralysis at Kurume University Hospital. When two or more EMG examinations were performed on the same subject, they were conducted at different stages of paralysis.

The muscles investigated were the vocalis (VOC), lateral cricoarytenoid (LCA), posterior cricoarytenoid (PCA), and cricothyroid (CT). In a few cases, the interarytenoid muscle (IA) was examined. Because it is innervated from the RLN bilaterally, it showed normal potentials, so that there was no need to examine it routinely. Because some patients were unable to tolerate the procedure, all four muscles were not examined in every case. Thus, the VOC was examined in 90, the LCA in 130, the PCA in 93, and the CT in 116 cases.

Bipolar needle electrodes were used. They were inserted into the laryngeal muscles transcutaneously (Hiroto, Hirano, Toyozumi, and Shin, 1962; Hirano and Ohala, 1969). EMG patterns were evaluated at several different locations in each muscle. In this way, the investigators could ensure that they had accounted for the phenomenon of different motor units in a given paralyzed muscle occasionally exhibiting different EMG patterns.

The EMG patterns obtained were related to the duration of paralysis, the position of the paretic vocal fold, the cause of paralysis, and the prognosis. Also, the EMG patterns were compared across the muscles investigated.

RESULTS AND DISCUSSION

The CT showed normal potentials in all but ten cases. Therefore, the results will be described primarily for the other three muscles with reference to the CT when the results are pertinent to the discussion.

Duration of Paralysis versus EMG Findings

There were six types of EMG patterns observed. These patterns will be referred to throughout the remainder of the chapter, and are as follows:

1. Electrical silence (S)
2. Fibrillation potentials (F)
3. Polyphasic potentials (P)
4. High amplitude potentials (H)
5. Normal potentials but reduced in number (n)
6. Normal potentials (N)

Table 20-1 shows the EMG patterns seen in the VOC, LCA, and PCA by the duration of the paralysis. Onset was determined by the reported time of trauma (e.g., endotracheal intubation or surgery) or the reported onset of hoarseness. When two or more different EMG patterns were observed within the same muscle, the categorization used in Table 20-1 was made according to the rules shown in Table 20-2.

All three muscles showed similar findings. Category F was noted at the earliest 12 days after the onset of paralysis and was also found in muscles paralyzed for more than one year. The earliest category P was observed was two months after onset and could be seen any time within one year after onset. In one case, P was observed at more than a year after onset. Category H was very rare, and when observed, occurred from 2 to 12 months after onset.

It should be noted that normal potentials (N or n) were found in many cases. The presence of normal potentials in the early stage indicates that the motor units in the recurrent laryngeal nerve were partly intact from the beginning of paralysis (incomplete paralysis) or that they had neuropraxia at the onset and had partly recovered by the time of the EMG examination.

TABLE 20-1.
EMG Patterns by Duration of Paralysis

Muscle	EMG Pattern	Duration of Paralysis							Total
		–2W	2W–1M	1M–2M	2M–3M	3M–6M	6M–12M	12M–	
VOC	S	0	3	1	1	2	3	6	16
	F	1	3	11	5	6	0	5	31
	P	0	0	0	1	4	2	0	7
	H	0	0	1	0	0	0	0	1
	N or n	3	3	15	2	5	4	3	35
	Total	4	9	28	9	17	9	14	90
LCA	S	1	2	0	0	3	2	3	11
	F	1	6	7	7	8	0	4	33
	P	0	0	0	3	6	5	1	15
	H	0	0	1	0	1	1	0	3
	N or n	2	8	25	5	9	6	13	68
	Total	4	16	33	15	27	14	21	130
PCA	S	0	2	0	0	3	2	6	13
	F	0	5	11	7	4	0	4	31
	P	0	0	0	1	0	3	0	4
	H	0	0	1	0	0	0	0	1
	N or n	2	3	14	4	5	7	9	44
	Total	2	10	26	12	12	12	19	93

The presence of normal potentials in a later stage indicates either an incomplete paralysis from the onset or regeneration of nerve fibers.

Table 20-3 shows the frequency of EMG categories for all 130 cases when the rules in Table 20-2 are applied to the three muscles. Electromyographic patterns S and F imply complete paralysis. Complete paralysis was noted in only 39 cases or 30 percent of the subjects sampled. As will be described later, 20 of the 130 cases had limited mobility and all 20 of these subjects showed some voluntary muscle action potentials.

TABLE 20-2.
Rules for Categorization When Two or More Different EMG Patterns Were Observed within the Same Muscle.

F + S → F
P + X → P
H + X → H
n + S, F or both → n
N + S, F or both → N

X: any pattern.

In the remaining 110 cases with a fixed vocal fold, complete paralysis accounted for 39 cases or 35 percent.

Differences in Vulnerability and Recovery

One of the questions addressed by the data presented here is whether or not there are any differences in vulnerability and recovery among the muscles studied. Since Semon (1881) first raised the issue many investigators have argued about potential differences but have been unable to draw conclusions from existing data. Results from the current study may shed some additional light on the topic.

Table 20-4 compares the frequency of EMG patterns among the three muscles studied. Categories P and H are included as one group in this table because both have the same clinical implication, namely, reinnervation. A chi square test was employed for statistical evaluation. There was no significant difference in frequency of EMG patterns among the muscles studied (Table 20-4A).

In order to investigate differences in vulnerability, comparisons were made for those cases seen within two months after onset (Table 20-4B). It was presumed that, within two months, no reinnervation had taken place, with only one exception. Therefore, any differences seen in EMG among the muscles could be attributed to differences in vulnerability. No significant difference, however, was determined among the three muscles.

In order to study differences in

TABLE 20-3.
Incidence of EMG Patterns in 130 Cases.

Silent	8
Fibrillation	31
Polyphasic	14
High amplitude	3
Normal (reduction of active units)	49
Normal*	25
Total	130

* 10 subjects showed evidence of misdirected reinnervation. The rule in Table 20-2 is applied when three muscles (VOC, LCA, and PCA) of the same subject presented different patterns.

TABLE 20-4.
Comparison of Frequency of EMG Patterns among VOC, LCA, and PCA.

A. Entire Cases

	S	F	P or H	n or N	Total
VOC	16 (18%)	31 (36%)	8 (9%)	35 (39%)	90
LCA	11 (8%)	33 (25%)	18 (14%)	68 (52%)	130
PCA	13 (14%)	31 (33%)	5 (5%)	44 (47%)	93
Total	40	85	31	147	313

$\chi^2 = 11.68 < 12.59 \ (= \chi_{0.05}^2)$

B. Early Cases (within 2 months)

	S	F	P or H	n or N	Total
VOC	4 (10%)	15 (37%)	1 (2%)	21 (51%)	41
LCA	3 (6%)	14 (26%)	1 (2%)	35 (66%)	53
PCA	2 (5%)	16 (42%)	1 (3%)	19 (50%)	38
Total	9	45	3	75	132

$\chi^2 = 4.78 < 12.59 \ (= \chi_{0.05}^2)$

C. Late Cases (after 2 months or later)

	S	F	P or H	n or N	Total
VOC	12 (24%)	16 (33%)	7 (14%)	14 (29%)	49
LCA	8 (10%)	19 (25%)	17 (22%)	33 (43%)	77
PCA	11 (20%)	15 (27%)	4 (7%)	25 (45%)	55
Total	31	50	28	72	181

$\chi^2 = 12.27 < 12.59 \ (= \chi_{0.05}^2)$

recovery among the muscles, a comparison was made for those cases classified as two months or more beyond the onset (Table 20-4C). Normal potentials in this period can come from those motor units that have not been denervated or from motor units that were denervated and had regenerated. As there were no differences evident in vulnerability among the muscles, if any differences exist among the muscles, they could be attributed to differences in recovery. The chi square test revealed no significant differences among the muscles.

Further analysis of intermuscle variations will be given. Of the 130 cases, 90 cases showed with the same EMG pattern in all muscles, whereas 40 cases showed different EMG patterns in different muscles. In 39 of these 40 cases it could be presumed, however, that if all the motor units in each muscle could have been studied, they all would have exhibited the same EMG pattern. For example, in some cases, one muscle showed n and F whereas the others showed F alone. In some other cases, one muscle exhibited n, P, and F whereas the others presented P and F or n and F.

There was an obvious difference in EMG between the VOC and the other muscles in only one case. This was a case seen 20 months after the paralysis developed following an upper respiratory infection. In this case, the VOC showed S, the LCA and CT showed N, and the PCA showed n. The vocal fold was fixed in the paramedian position and was markedly atrophic. One can presume that, in this case, almost all motor units in the VOC failed to reinnervate, whereas many motor units in the LCA and PCA were reinnervated. It was difficult to determine whether CT was involved.

It should be kept in mind that EMG can not determine the ratio of the number of normally innervated motor units to that of the entire motor unit pool. It is highly probable that this ratio differs from muscle to muscle in cases of recurrent laryngeal nerve paralysis. In exceptional cases, the ratio difference may be great enough to be observable by EMG, as in the case reported here.

In summary, in the present series there were no systematic differences in vulnerability or recovery among the muscles studied. Although the ratio of the number of normally innervated motor units to the entire motor unit pool differs from muscle to muscle, this

difference is generally not reflected in EMG recording. For clinical purposes, EMG recordings of the VOC and CT are generally sufficient in cases of laryngeal paralysis.

Location of Paretic Vocal Fold versus EMG Findings

During the last century there have been numerous discussions of the relevance of the position of the paretic vocal fold. The discussions have grouped around two historical hypotheses: ''the Semon-Rosenbach law'' and 'the Wagner-Grossmann theory''; both of which, in modern laryngology, have been determined to be irrelevant (Hiroto, 1966; Hirose, 1970; Sawashima, 1984). Therefore, rather than repeat these discussions, the current paper will focus on determining whether there are any relevant relationships between the location of the paretic vocal fold and EMG findings.

By mirror examination, the paretic vocal fold exhibited limited movements in 20 cases, was fixed in the median position in 22 cases, was fixed in the paramedian position in 78 cases, and was fixed in the intermediate position in 10 cases. Table 20-5 shows the relationship between the location of the paretic vocal fold and EMG findings. In Table 20-5, EMG patterns are divided into two major groups: S and F are put together in one group and P, H, n, and N are in the other group. The former group implies absence of voluntary action potentials or innervated motor units, whereas the latter consists of cases with voluntary action potentials.

TABLE 20-5.
Relationship Between EMG Finding and Position of Paretic Vocal Fold. (Numbers in Parentheses Indicate Numbers of Cases in which CT was Involved.)

A. VOC

	S or F	P, H, n, or N	Total
Limited mobility	1(8%)	12(92%)	13
Median	5(38%)	8(62%)	13
Paramedian	34(63%)	20(37%)	54
Fixed	(7)		
Intermediate	7(70%)	3(30%)	10
	(2)		
Total	46(60%)	31(40%)	77

For fixed cases, $\chi^2 = 3.12 < 5.99 \, (= \chi_{0.05}^2)$

B. LCA

	S or F	P, H, n, or N	Total
Limited mobility	1(5%)	19(95%)	20
Median	5(23%)	17(77%)	22
Paramedian	34(44%)	44(56%)	78
Fixed	(6)	(2)	
Intermediate	4(40%)	6(60%)	10
	(2)		
Total	43(31%)	67(69%)	110

For fixed cases, $\chi^2 = 3.14 < 5.99 \, (= \chi_{0.05}^2)$

C. PCA

	S or F	P, H, n, or N	Total
Limited mobility	1(6%)	16(94%)	17
Median	5(42%)	7(58%)	12
Paramedian	33(58%)	24(42%)	57
Fixed	(6)		
Intermediate	5(71%)	2(29%)	7
	(2)		
Total	43(57%)	33(43%)	76

For fixed cases, $\chi^2 = 1.76 < 5.99 \, (= \chi_{0.05}^2)$

D. Entire Three Muscles

	S or F	P, H, n, or N	Total
Limited mobility	0	20	20
Median	5(23%)	17(77%)	22
Paramedian	31(40%)	47(60%)	78
Fixed	(6)	(2)	
Intermediate	3(30%)	7(70%)	10
	(2)		
Total	39(35%)	71(65%)	110

For fixed cases, $\chi^2 = 2.33 < 5.99 \, (= \chi_{0.05}^2)$

Cases With Limited Mobility

All 20 of the cases with limited vocal fold movements showed voluntary action potentials in at least two of the three muscles investigated. Twelve of these cases showed restricted abduction. The vocal fold adducted to the midline but did not abduct beyond the intermediate position. In 11 of these 12 cases, EMG was obtained from both the abductors and the adductors. Signs of denervation were partially evident in three cases. The etiology of paralysis varied: heart surgery in one, endotracheal intubation in one, a cold in three, and unknown in six cases. The EMG findings coupled with the etiologies indicate that no complete section of the nerve took place in any of the cases. EMG findings concerning differences in motor unit involvement of the adductors and abductors were as follows: In two cases, EMG indicated that more motor units were innervated in the adductors than in the abductors, whereas in the other nine, EMG did not demonstrate any obvious differences between the two.

Cases With Fixed Vocal fold

In the 110 cases with a fixed vocal fold, it appeared that the more medially the paretic vocal fold was located, the more often were voluntary action potentials observed. The chi square test, however, did not reveal a significant relationship between the location of the paretic vocal fold and the EMG findings.

In Table 20-5, the number of cases that showed abnormal EMG patterns in the CT are indicated in parentheses. There was a total of ten cases in which the CT was involved. In eight of the ten, the paretic fold was fixed in the paramedian position, whereas it was in the intermediate position in the other two. There were no cases in which the vocal fold was fixed in the median position. Of the ten cases with CT involvement, eight showed S or F in the VOC, LCA, and PCA as well as in the CT. In the other two, one case exhibited P in the LCA and CT, and the other case showed n in the LCA and CT.

The contribution of the CT to the position of the paretic vocal fold can be best illustrated in the cases of complete paralysis. Table 20-6 shows the relationship between the position of the paretic fold and CT involvement. There was a tendency that the more lateral the vocal fold, the more frequently the CT was involved. The chi square test, however, revealed no significant relationship between the position of paretic vocal fold and CT involvement.

Etiology of Paralysis versus EMG Findings

As described earlier, incomplete paralysis was frequent in the present series. Table 20-7 shows the EMG findings by the etiology of the presenting paralysis.

As can be seen from this table, in those cases within two months after onset where no reinnervation had taken place, normal potentials were significantly more frequent for paralysis caused by a cold and that of unknown etiology. No significant differences were observed for paralysis due to other etiologies.

TABLE 20-6.

Relationship Between Vocal Fold Position and CT Involvement in Cases of Complete Paralysis Where EMG Showed S or F in all Muscles.

Vocal Fold Position	CT		Total
	Involved	Not Involved	
Median	0	5	5
Paramedian	6	25	31
Intermediate	2	1	3
Total	8	31	39

TABLE 20-7.

EMG Findings by Etiology of Paralysis

Etiology	Normal Potentials in EMG		Total
	Present	Absent	
Neck tumor	0	1	1
Neck surgery	6	4(1)	10(1)
Neck trauma	1	0	1
Endotracheal intubation	2	2	4
Chest diseases	0	0	0
Chest surgery	2	1	3
Cold	13	2(1)	15(1)
Unknown	15(1)	4(1)	19(2)
Total	39(1)	14(3)	53(4)

Numbers in parentheses indicate number of patients with CT involved.

Late Cases (after 2 months)

Etiology	Voluntary Action Potentials (P, H, n, N)		Total
	Present	Absent	
Neck tumor	1	0	1
Neck surgery	2	3(2)	5(2)
Neck trauma	3	1	4
Endotracheal intubation	0	0	0
Chest diseases	2	3	5
Chest surgery	3	2	5
Cold	19(1)	11(2)	30(3)
Unknown	22	5(1)	27(1)
Total	52(1)	25(5)	77(6)

Numbers in parentheses indicate number of patients with CT involved.

In the cases two months or more after onset where reinnervation could have taken place, cases with voluntary action potentials were significantly more frequent than those without voluntary action potentials for paralysis of unknown etiology. No significant difference was found for paralysis from other etiologies.

Prognosis of laryngeal nerve palsy caused by a cold or of unknown etiology has been reported to be generally favorable (Hirano, Ohno, Nagashima, and Maeyama, 1970; Nozoe, Hirano, Shin, and Maeyama, 1972). The results of the present study indicate that the favorable prognosis can be attributed to the incomplete paralysis often present in these groups.

CT involvement occurred only in those cases of paralysis caused by neck surgery, colds, or unknown etiology.

Prognostic Issues

Prognosis of Paralysis

From a clinical point of view, one of the most important issues in unilateral recurrent laryngeal nerve paralysis is prognosis. Of the series reported here, 61 cases were followed for one year or more after the onset of paralysis. The prognosis of paralysis will be discussed in relation to the EMG findings of these 61 cases.

Sixteen of the 61 cases had some mobility at the time of the EMG recording. All of these 16 cases showed normal potentials. Further recovery, however, was mixed: nine recovered completely, one showed inprovement but

not complete recovery, and six remained unchanged.

Table 20-8 shows prognosis in relation to EMG findings in the 45 cases that had a fixed vocal fold at the time of the EMG recording. These data indicate that the most important factor in EMG, for prognostic purposes, was the presence of action potentials induced by voluntary activity. Although the number of cases was too small for statistical evaluations, the following tendencies were noted in Table 20-8:

1. In cases examined within six months after onset, the recovery rate was higher for those cases that showed voluntary action potentials (12/19) than those cases that had none (2/10).

2. The position of the paretic vocal fold appeared to be important for prognosis in the period of three to six months after onset. All four cases with the paretic fold in the median position recovered mobility, but all four cases with the paretic fold in the paramedian position failed to recover mobility.

3. EMG was not useful for prognostic purposes after six months following onset, because none of these recovered mobility regardless of EMG findings.

Prognosis of Hoarseness

The prognosis of hoarseness was subjectively evaluated by the patients. The evaluation was made one year or more after the onset and categorized in three groups: (1) voice recovered normally, (2) voice improved but not to his/her normal level, and (3) voice remained unchanged.

TABLE 20-8.
Relationship Between EMG Findings and Prognosis of Paralysis

Duration	Vocal Fold Position	Voluntary Action Potentials	
		Absent	**Present**
−1M	Median		2/2
	Paramedian	1/2 }1/2	1/2 }4/5
	Intermediate		1/1
1–2M	Median		0/1
	Paramedian	02 }0/2	2/3 }2/4
	Intermediate		
2–3M	Median	0/1	1/1
	Paramedian	0/2 }0/3	1/1 }2/2
	Intermediate		
3–6M	Median	0/1	4/4
	Paramedian	1/2 }1/3	0/4 }4/8
	Intermediate		
6M–	Median		0/1
	Paramedian	0/7 }0/8	0/6 }0/8
	Intermediate	0/1	0/1

Denominator: number of cases in each category; Numerator: number of cases that recovered mobility.

Data were obtained from 81 cases. Of the 81, 18 had some mobility of the paretic fold and normal potentials at the time of EMG. Discussion will focus on the remaining 63 cases with fixed vocal fold at the time of EMG. No voice therapy was given to any cases. The results are shown in Table 20-9.

Unlike the prognosis for vocal fold mobility, the prognosis for voice improvement, as assessed by the patient, did not show any consistent relationship to EMG findings. Regardless of EMG findings, complete recovery of voice did not take place in the cases six months or more after onset.

In 56 of the 81 cases, data were obtained for both mobility and voice. The relationship between prognosis for mobility and that for voice is shown in Table 20-10. There was good agreement between the mobility and voice recovery in many cases (40/56). In 12 cases, voice was improved without recovery of mobility. There were no cases, however, in which recovery of mobility was not associated with an improvement of voice. Thus, when EMG indicates a possibility of recovery of vocal fold mobility, one can also expect an improvement of voice. When EMG indicates a poor prognosis

TABLE 20-9.
Relationship Between EMG Findings and Prognosis of Hoarseness

Duration	Vocal Fold Position	Voluntary Action Potentials							
		Absent				Present			
		Norm.	Imp.	Unch.	Total	Norm.	Imp.	Unch.	Total
-1M	Med.	1			1	1			1
	Para.	2	1		3	2	1	1	4
	Int.				0	1			1
1-2M	Med.				0			1	1
	Para.		1	1	2	4	4		8
	Int.				0				0
2-3M	Med.	1	1		2		1		1
	Para.	1	1	1	3	1			1
	Int.		1		1				
3-6M	Med.			1	1	3	1		4
	Para.	3	2		5		2	2	4
	Int.			1	1	1			1
6M-	Med.						1		1
	Para.			7	7		3	4	7
	Int.			1	1		1	1	2

Med.: Median; Para.: Paramedian; Int.: Intermediate; Norm.: Normal; Imp.: Improved; Unch.: Unchanged.

for mobility, voice may or may not recover within six months after the onset.

COMMENTS

Thus far we have presented results and discussion without reference to the pertinent literature. In the final section of this paper we will attempt to integrate our findings with the existent literature.

EMG Patterns Observed In Laryngeal Paralysis

In human skeletal muscles, insertion fibrillation potentials ap-pear 8 to 14 days and spontaneous fibrillation potentials appear 2 to 4 weeks following denervation (Mayo Clinic, 1964). In laryngeal muscles, fibrillation potentials have been reported as early as 22 days (Hiroto, Hirano, and Tomita, 1968) and 30 days (Ueda, 1968) after onset. In the present study, fibrillation potentials were observed as early as 12 days after onset, which is considerably earlier than previously reported for laryngeal muscles, but consistent with reports for skeletal muscles. Thus, one can say that the time of appearance of fibrillation potentials in laryngeal paralysis does not differ signifi-

TABLE 20-10.
Relationship Between Prognosis for Mobility and That for Voice

Mobility	Voice			Total
	Normal	Improved	Unchanged	
Complete recovery	16	1		17
Incomplete recovery	3	9		12
No recovery	2	10	15	27
Total	21	20	15	56

cantly from that in paralysis of skeletal muscles.

The time of appearance of polyphasic potentials depends on the distance from the site of injury to the muscle. Ueda (1968) investigated 56 cases of RLN paralysis caused by thyroid surgery, and found polyphasic potentials as early as 50 days after onset. The site of injury in Ueda's cases was close to the muscles. In a study conducted by Hiroto and colleagues (1968), polyphasic potentials were recorded in cases six weeks to six months after onset. In the present study, they were found at the earliest two months after onset. On the basis of these data, one can say that the earliest reinnervation of denervated laryngeal muscles takes place at approximately 50 days after onset of paralysis.

High amplitude potentials are rare (Hiroto et al., 1968; Ueda, 1968). Normal potentials were reported in early stages of paralysis (Hiroto et al., 1968; Ueda, 1968). Following denervation, the earliest appearance of normal potentials induced by regenerated axons is approximately 80 days after onset (Ueda, 1968).

Vulnerability and Recovery

Since Semon (1881) first reported that motor fibers innervating the PCA were more vulnerable than the motor fibers for the adductor muscles, numerous pro and con arguments have been made. Negus (1962) agreed with Semon in terms of the greater vulnerability of the abductor muscle from an evolutionary point of view. This viewpoint was supported by Arnold (1957), Sawashima (1958), and Hirose (1968).

When the abductor muscle alone is paralyzed, the vocal fold moves between the median and the intermediate position but is not abducted beyond the intermediate position. Such cases have been reported by Arnold (1957), Sawashima, Sato, Funasaka, and Totsuka (1958), Ueda (1968), and Hiroto and colleagues (1968). Ueda (1968) followed the course of recovery in 35 cases of recurrent laryngeal nerve paralysis caused by thyroid surgery. The paralysis in these cases was presumably neuropraxia because no fibrillation potentials were observed by EMG. Ueda reported a proclivity for the paretic fold to take the following course: intermediate position →

paramedian position → median position → limited movement with abduction restricted → normal movement. In his EMG study, the LCA tended to recover sooner than the VOC and PCA. He recorded EMG in six cases at the time of restricted abduction and found that in five of them, normally activated motor units were fewer in the PCA than in the LCA.

In experimental studies with dogs, the abductor muscle tended to be affected sooner than the adductor muscles and recovery tended to take place in the adductors sooner than in the abductor when the nerve received gradual mechanical stress such as pressure. However, when the nerve was affected by cold temperature or drugs, no consistent differences in vulnerability and recovery were noted between the two groups of muscles (Kawano, 1964; Ohyama, Ueda, Harvey, Mogi, and Ogura, 1972).

Originally, "Semon's law" was based on a gradually progressing paralysis. On the basis of both clinical and experimental studies described earlier, we presume that the greater vulnerability of the abductor occurs in gradually progressing paralysis and the more rapid recovery of the adductor muscles holds true only with selected cases of neuropraxia.

The present series included paralysis from different etiologies. This may explain why we were unable to find significant differences in vulnerability and recovery among the muscles. It is obvious from our data that "Semon's law" on vulnerability is applicable only to selected cases of recurrent laryngeal nerve palsy. In the present series, 12 cases exhibited restricted abduction. Although a dominant involvement of the abductor over the adductors was demonstrated with EMG in only two cases, we presume it was present in all 12 cases, because EMG is not always capable of demonstrating quantitative differences in the number of motor units.

Position of Paretic Vocal Fold

Complete paralysis, that is, a complete blockade of impulse conduction of all the motor units, does not often occur in the larynx (Faaborg-Andersen, 1957; Hirose et al., 1967; Hiroto et al., 1968; Ueda, 1968; Blair, Berry, and Briant, 1978). This is also true in the present series. Both the "Semon-Rosenbach law" and the "Wagner-Grossmann theory" appear to be premised on a complete paralysis of each muscle. For this and other reasons, it is not meaningful to discuss the two hypotheses in a clinical context.

Some relationships between the position of the paretic vocal fold and the degree of incomplete paralysis have been demonstrated by Ueda (1968) and Hirose and colleagues (1967). These authors observed that the fewer the paralyzed motor units, the more medial was the paretic fold located. In the present series, this relationship was not statistically significant. However, the more favorable prognosis in the median compared to the paramedian position of the paretic cord appears to support the results of Ueda and Hirose and colleagues.

Hirose and his co-workers also demonstrated a tendency for a more laterally located vocal fold with involvement of the CT. In the present series, involvement of the CT was not significantly related to the location of the fixed vocal fold.

The location of the paretic vocal fold depends not only on the balance of tonus of the intrinsic laryngeal muscles, but also on anatomical factors, including the location and morphology of the cricoarytenoid joint. The location of the vocal fold in cadavers differs greatly from individual to individual (Mukasa and Ueda, 1962). It is impossible to tell, on the basis of the location of the paretic fold alone, whether the CT is involved or not.

Prognostic Aspects

The significance of EMG for prognostic purposes in laryngeal paralysis has not been closely investigated. In skeletal muscles, EMG from denervated muscles shows the following consistent changes in pattern along the course of spontaneous recovery: electrical silence → fibrillation potentials → polyphasic potentials → high amplitude potentials → normal potentials. Recovery of muscular function takes place following reinnervation.

The present study demonstrated that in laryngeal paralysis, a good prognosis is usually associated with incomplete paralysis affecting a part of the motor unit pool or neuropraxia. In Ueda's report (1968) on paralysis following thyroid surgery, those cases that recovered mobility were presumed to be neuropraxia because they did not show signs of axon degeneration with EMG. Clinically

then, the most important purposes of EMG are to determine (1) whether the motor units are involved entirely or partially, and (2) whether the paralysis is due to neuropraxia or to degeneration of the axons.

Traditionally, clinicians have waited for one year before determining if surgical intervention for unilateral laryngeal paralysis is indicated. It is, however, a waste of valuable time to wait for spontaneous recovery in those cases with a poor prognosis, especially for professional voice users. EMG provides valuable information in determining this prognosis. Etiology and duration of palsy, location of the paretic vocal fold, and stroboscopic findings (Hirano, Shin, and Nozoe, 1977) provide the clinician with a combination that increases the accuracy of prognosis.

When the prognosis is considered to be favorable, we recommend voice therapy. When the prognosis is presumed to be unfavorable in cases within six months after onset, intrafold injection of temporary augmentation materials is recommended. For cases with a poor prognosis six months or more after the onset, intrafold injection of a permanent material or surgical mediofixation is recommended.

CONCLUSIONS

The results of the present study integrated with data in existing literature led us to the following conclusions:

1. In many patients with laryngeal paralysis, the motor units are not totally involved, and the diagnosis should be incomplete paralysis.

2. The time of appearance of fibrillation and polyphasic potentials following denervation of laryngeal muscles is almost identical to that of skeletal muscles.

3. Greater vulnerability of the abductor than the adductors seems to occur only in selected cases of gradually progressing paralysis.

4. A more rapid recovery of the adductors than the abductor seems to occur in certain cases of neuropraxia.

5. There is a tendency for the paretic vocal fold to lie more medially when fewer motor units are affected.

6. CT involvement cannot be determined by the location of the paretic vocal fold.

7. EMG is useful for prognosis in paralysis of six months or less. The presence of voluntary action potentials is the most favorable prognostic sign.

REFERENCES

Arnold, G.E. (1957). Vocal rehabilitation of paralytic dysphonia; III Present concept of laryngeal paralysis. *Arch Otolaryngol, 65*, 317–336.

Blair, R.L., Berry, H., and Briant, T.D R. (1978). Laryngeal electromyography: Technique and application. *Otolaryngologic Clinics of North America, 11*, 325–346.

Faaborg-Andersen, K. (1957). Electromyographic investigation of intrinsic laryngeal muscles in humans. *Acta Physiol Scand, 41*, 9–148.

Hirano, M., Nozoe, I., Shin, T., and Maeyama, T. (1974). Electromyographic findings in recurrent laryngeal nerve paralysis. A study of 130 cases. *Practice Otologia Kyoto, 67*, 231–242.

Hirano, M., and Ohala, J. (1969). Use of hooked-wire electrodes for electromyography of the intrinsic laryngeal muscles. *J Speech Hearing Res, 12*, 362–373.

Hirano, M., Ohno, T., Nagashima, T., and Maeyama, T. (1970). Prognostic aspects of hoarseness in recurrent laryngeal nerve paralysis. *J Otolaryngol Jpn, 73*, 892–899.

Hirano, M., Shin, T., and Nozoe, I. (1977). Prognostic aspects of recurrent laryngeal nerve paralysis. *IALPs 17th International Congress of Logopedics and Phoniatrics* (pp. 96–103). Copenhagen.

Hirose, H. (1970). Recurrent laryngeal nerve paralysis. In T. Kitamura (Ed.), *Recent Advances in Otorhinolaryngology* (pp. 528–542). Tokyo: Ishiyaku Press.

Hirose, H., Kobayashi, T., Okamura, M., Kurauchi, Y., Iwamura, S., Ushijima, T., and Sawashima, M. (1967). Recurrent laryngeal nerve palsy. *J Otolaryngol Jpn, 70*, 1–17.

Hiroto, I. (1966). The mechanism of phonation. Pathophysiological aspects of the larynx. *Practica Otologia Kyoto, 39*, 229–291.

Hiroto, I., Hirano, M., Toyozumi, Y., and Shin, T. (1962). A new method of placement of a needle electrode in the intrinsic laryngeal muscles for electromyography. Insertion through the skin. *Practica Otologia Kyoto, 55*, 499–504.

Hiroto, I., Hirano, M., and Tomita, H. (1968). Electromyographic investigation of human vocal cord paralysis. *Ann. Otol. Rhinol. Laryngol., 77*, 296–304.

Kawano, Y. (1964). Study on laryngeal paralysis. *J Otolaryngol Jpn, 67*, 159–176.

Mayo Clinic. (1964). *Clinical examination in neurology*. Philadelphia: Saunders.

Mukasa, T., and Ueda, T. (1962). The position of the vocal cords in cadaver and so-called cadaveric position of the vocal cords. *J Otolaryngol Jpn, 65*, 184–192.

Negus, V.E. (1962). *The comparative anatomy and physiology of the larynx*. New York: Hafner Publishing Co.

Nozoe, I., Hirano, M., Shin, T., and Maeyama, T. (1972). Recurrent laryngeal nerve palsy. A clinical study of 400 cases. *Otologia Fukuoka, 18*, 411–417.

Ohyama, M., Ueda, N., Harvey, J.E., Mogi, G., and Ogura, J.H. (1972). Electrophysiologic study of reinnervated laryngeal motor units. *Laryngoscope, 132*, 237–251.

Sawashima, M. (1958). Some consideration on the paralysis of the recurrent laryngeal nerve. *Oto-Rhino-Laryngology Tokyo, 1*, 448–452.

Sawashima, M. (1984). Hypotheses on position of vocal fold. In H. Ishii (Ed.), *Recurrent laryngeal nerve paralysis* (pp. 59–67). Bunkodo: Tokyo.

Sawashima, M., Sato, M., Funasaka, S., and Totsuka, G. (1958). Electromyographic study of the human larynx and its clinical application. *J Otolaryngol Jpn, 61*, 1357–1364.

Semon, F. (1881). Clinical remarks on the proclivity of the abductor fibers of the recurrent laryngeal nerve to become affected sooner than the abductor fibers, or even exclusively, in cases of undoubted central or peripheral injury or disease of the roots or trunks of the pneumogastric, spinal accessory, or recurrent nerves. *Archives of Laryngology, 2*, 197–222.

Ueda, N. (1968). A clinical study of the recurrent laryngeal nerve paralysis following surgical operations. Part II. *Hiroshima Medical Journal, 16*, 431–459.

CHAPTER 21

Idiopathic Associated Laryngeal Palsy

Noriko K. NISHIZAWA
and Hajime HIROSE

"Associated laryngeal palsy" is a complex syndrome in which the larynx is involved along with other neurological disorders. Historically, eponymous nomenclature was applied to various combinations of cranial nerve disorders (Cody, 1946). An enormous number of reports have described various etiologies, both central and peripheral: neoplastic, vascular, and degenerative diseases (Hirose, 1984). Additionally, there is a concept of "idiopathic" laryngeal palsy, a diagnosis made in the absence of any specific etiology. As is the case with Bell's palsy, in idiopathic recurrent nerve palsy the origin and etiology remain unknown.

CASE STUDIES

Table 21-1 summarizes the results of a survey of the causes of associated laryngeal palsy in 40 clinical cases observed over the last ten years at the Voice and Speech Clinic, University of Tokyo Hospital. Motor neuron disease was excluded from this study because of its exceptional clinical course and pathogenesis (Hirose, 1984). In 11 cases, intracranial lesions such as tumors, degenerative diseases of the central nervous system, and cerebrovascular diseases were found to have produced the palsy. In nine cases, extracranial lesions were suspected. In the remaining 21 cases, the pathogenesis remained unknown even after exhaustive examination, and the diagnosis of idopathic associated laryngeal palsy was made.

The clinical features of the 21 cases with idiopathic associated laryngeal palsy are shown in Table 21-2. All patients were over 30 years of age. There was no preponderence of either sex. Some characteristic features of

249

TABLE 21-1.
Cause of Associated Laryngeal Palsy in 40 Cases

Intracranial tumor	3
Operation for intracranial tumor	2
Extracranial tumor	1
Operation for extracranial tumor	5
Syringobulbia	2
Cerebrovascular disease	3
Sarcoidosis	1
Trauma	2
Idiopathic	21
Total	40

neurological symptoms were identified: (1) The palsy was unilateral in 20 cases. Symmetrical paralysis was not observed in any case included in this study. In 15 cases, the palsies were restricted to the lower cranial nerves: glossopharyngeal, vagal, accessory, and hypoglossal. Of the other six cases, three showed palsies of the lower cranial and facial nerves; one showed palsy of the lower cranial, facial, and motor fibers of the trigeminal nerve; and in the remaining two, diffuse symptoms of upper and lower cranial nerve involvement developed. (2) Dysfunctions of the motor fibers predominated in all the cases. Pure motor paralysis was seen in 18 cases. Minor sensory symptoms such as hemifacial paresthesia were observed in three patients. Pyramidal tract signs and cerebellar symptoms were noted in two patients.

As antecedent events, acute upper respiratory infections and irritable pain around the temporal region were noticed in several cases. In one patient, an operation under lumbar anesthesia preceded the onset of the palsy. The onset was acute or subacute in 16 cases in which the palsy became complete within one week. In the other five patients, the palsies relapsed or developed gradually over many years.

Recovery was noted within several months in 11 cases. Six patients showed no recovery after a year-long follow-up. The remaining four patients were lost to follow-up, so that information on return of function is unknown.

DISCUSSION

The present series cannot be considered clinically homogeneous. Idiopathic associated laryngeal palsy in this study may correspond to those syndromes reported under the name of polyneuritis cranialis (Toyokura, 1959; Konodo et al., 1963) or multiple cranial neuritis (Kawamura et al., 1973). As for cranial polyneuropathy of unknown etiology, Toyokura (1959) has stated that (1) polyneuritis cranialis is not a single disease entity but a syndrome; and (2) polyneuritis cranialis is a neuropathy that primarily involves multiple cranial nerves, is almost always symmetrical, and

TABLE 21-2.
Clinical Manifestations of the 21 Cases of Idiopathic Associated Laryngeal Palsy

case	age/sex	III	IV	VI (eye)	V jaw	VII face	X s.p.	v.f.	ct	XI	XII	V sensory	cerebellar	pyramidal
1	61 F					l	l							
2	53 F					r	r	?						
3	36 M					l	l	?						
4	34 M					l	l	l	l					
5	62 F					r	r	r	r					
6	67 M					l	l	l	l					
7	62 M					r	r	r	r					+
8	41 F					l	l							+
9	78 F					l	l	?			l			
10	33 F					l	l	l			l			
11	61 M				rl		r	r						
12	64 F	r	r	r	r	r	r	r	r	r		r		
13	38 M	l	l	l		l	l	l	?	l				l
14	67 F					l	l	l	l					
15	32 F					r	r	r						
16	43 M				l		l	l	l					
17	64 M						l	l	l	l				
18	54 F						l	l		l	l			
19	40 F						l	l	?	l				
20	32 M				l	l	l							
21	69 M					r	r	r	r	r	r			

s.p.; soft palate, v.c.; vocal fold, c.t.; cricothyroid muscle
r; right, l; left, rl; bilateral, ?; not examined

other manifestations	case no.
1. antecedent event	
cold	3,4,5, 10,11, 20
pain around the ear	3,4, 7, 13, 16
operation	17
2. clinical course	
acute evolution	1,2,3,4,5,6,7,8,9 14,15,16,17,18,19,20
recovery	1, 3,4,5,6,7,8 16,17, 19,20
recurrent	10,11,12,13, 21

may occur with or without slight neurological signs involving the limbs and trunk. Because the etiology of these syndromes remains unestablished (Arnason, 1975), we should avoid subdividing or unifying these cases according to hypothetical pathogeneses (Toyokura, 1959; Konodo et al., 1963). Nonetheless, it might be re-warding to analyze the clinical features of these cases from an etiological aspect with special reference to several neurological disorders reported in the literature.

Guillain-Barré Syndrome

Guillain-Barré syndrome is an acutely, or subacutely, evolving paralytic disease of unestablished etiology with acellular hyper-albuminosis of the cerebrospinal fluid (CSF) (Hirayama, 1974). The palsy may be confined to the cranial nerves without involvement of the other peripheral nerves (Ando et al., 1975). In a broad sense, all of the cases in the present study could be included in this syndrome or its subtypes (Konodo et al., 1963; Kawamura et al., 1973). However, the clinical manifestations of the present cases were not strictly compatible with those of the typical Guillain-Barré syndrome. Table 21-3 presents a comparison between the typical Guillan-Barré syndrome (Sobue, 1974) and the present series of cases. As can be seen in the table, the typical clinical course of the Guillain-Barré syndrome is rather uniform. In our study, 13 cases (Number 1, 3, 4, 5, 6, 9, 14, 15, 16, 17, 18, 19, and 20), showed an acute development, benign prognosis, and pure motor paralysis without long tract signs. They were thought to meet the criteria of this syndrome. The other eight cases could be differentiated from this typical syndrome by the chronic or progressive course of their disease and by complications in the long tract or cerebellum.

In several of the 13 cases compatible with the Guillain-Barré syndrome, we noticed antecedent events of acute upper respiratory infection or irritable pain around the temporal region, both of which are known to be common in the Guillain-Barré syndrome. In spite of these similarities, there were differences in age distribution (Araki, 1974; Sobue, 1974) and sex preponderence (Wiederholt et al., 1964; Sobue, 1974). In particular, the palsies in our 13 cases were

restricted to the unilateral cranial nerves caudal to the trigeminal nerve, whereas in the Guillain-Barré syndrome, symmetrical palsies are common (Cody, 1946; Osler et al, 1960; Ando et al., 1975; Shibata et al., 1975).

There seems to be general agreement concerning the participation of an aberrant immune response in the pathogenesis of the Guillain-Barré syndrome (Igata et al., 1974; Arnason, 1975). On the other hand, Nozoe and colleagues (1974) have reported three cases of unilateral lower cranial nerve palsy under the diagnosis of polyneuritis cranialis, while suspecting the participation of a viral infection. On the basis of polyneuropathies that resemble Guillain-Barré syndrome restricted to the lower cranial nerves of one side, it has been suggested that not only systemic reactions such as allergy, but also local factors such as viral infection may play an important role in the pathogenesis of this syndrome.

Viral Infection of the Cranial Nerves

Herpes zoster and herpes simplex viruses are regarded as being causative agents in peripheral nerve palsy (Hirose, 1984). Accumulating information points to common modes of behavior of these viruses within the peripheral nervous system (Baringer et al., 1975).

Hunt (1907) has suggested that herpes zoster invasion of the geniculate ganglion might be responsible for the complications of herpes zoster oticus and the involvement of the seventh and

TABLE 21-3.
Comparison Between the Typical Manifestation of the Guillain-Barré Syndrome and the Present Cases

	Guillain-Barré syndrome 26 cases from Sobue (1974)	Present study 21 cases
Under 30 years old	62%	0%
Rate for male patients	77%	48%
Acute evolution within several weeks	100%	76%
Recovery within several months	100%	67%
Antecedent event	88%	29%
Motor palsy dominant	100%	100%
Bilateral	100%	10%
Acellular hyperalbuminosis of CSF	100%	—
Long tract or cerebellar sign	0%	10%

eighth cranial nerves. Further, he has pointed out that herpetic lesions of the ganglia of the glossopharyngeal and vagal nerves might be responsible for herpes zoster oticus by transmission via Arnold's nerve (Hunt, 1910). Engstrom and colleagues (1949) and Font (1952) have suggested that because the region of the auricle and external auditory canal is supplied by the 5th, 7th, 9th, 10th, and the upper cervical spinal nerves, it is possible for paralysis of the facial nerve to occur as a result of zosterian inflammatory involvement from the ganglion of any of these nerves. Font (1952) has further reported "zoster sine herpete" (Lewis, 1958) and suggested that idiopathic associated laryngeal palsy might be the result of viral infection. These historical discussions are suggestive of the possibility of a peripheral pathway for viral invasion of the lower cranial nerves. Except for two cases with oculomotor palsies, most of the neurological symptoms in the other cases are explainable by viral transmission through the previously mentioned peripheral pathways and through the ansa hypoglossi pathway.

Recent studies have implicated the herpes simplex virus as a causative agent in Bell's palsy (McCormick, 1972). Adour (1976) and Djupesland and colleagues (1977) have suggested that some reactivating stimulus such as a cold can activate latent viruses in the ganglion cells and produce cranial polyneuritis. Djupesland and colleagues (1977) have suggested not only peripheral but also central pathways for the transmission of the virus.

In the present cases, herpetic vesicles diagnostic of herpes infection were not found. In serological study, cases 1, 9, and 21 showed an especially high titer suggesting a relapsing neuritis caused by herpes simplex virus.

Other viruses such as influenza A2 (Ishii et al., 1971), influenza B (Sato et al., 1981), and adenovirus (Wells, 1971) have been suspected of being responsible for peripheral neuritis, especially for recurrent nerve palsy. It is still debatable whether these viruses invade the peripheral nerves directly, or act as a trigger for a systemic reaction such as a neuro-allergy.

Brainstem Encephalitis

In the nucleus ambiguus, the motoneuron pools of the individual muscles have a topographic distribution in relation to one another, rather than being randomly intermingled (Lawn, 1966; Yoshida et al., 1982). Consequently, selective palsy of individual muscles can result from localized intranuclear lesions, as in the case of bulbar poliomyelitis (Wyke et al., 1976).

Under the diagnosis of brainstem encephalitis, Möller (1956) has reported 40 cases of unilateral lower cranial nerve palsy with antecedent events of upper respiratory infection or irritable pain in the temporal region. All showed an acute onset and benign prognosis. He considers the origin of the palsy to have been a focal lesion in the lower brainstem for the following reasons: (1) the injury was unilateral, whereas neuritis and radiculitis often cause bilateral symmetrical paresis; (2) dissociated paresis, such as paresis of only the vocal fold function of the Xth nerve, indicated nuclear, paranuclear, or intranuclear injury rather than injury to the nerve fibers; and (3) mild symptoms of other conduction tracts, especially of the pyramidal tract, occurred in many cases. Histopathological evidence of degenerative change in the brainstem with little change in the peripheral nerves has been reported by Arima and colleagues (1962) in the autopsy of a patient with acute cranial nerve palsy. Viral infection (Arima et al., 1962;

Djupesland et al., 1977; Ellison et al., 1977) and allergic reaction (Arima et al., 1962) have been suggested as etiological factors in brainstem encephalitis. It is sometimes difficult to distinguish clinically between central and peripheral injury, especially in cases without signs of central nervous system involvement (Vernet, 1918; Moeller, 1956; Arima et al., 1962). In fact, most recent reports on brainstem encephalitis have suggested complications of the central nervous system such as ataxia (Arima et al., 1962; Ogawa et al., 1969; Iwasa et al., 1975). In the present cases, acute inflammatory lesions in the brainstem were suspected in cases 7 and 8 with long tract and cerebellar signs. Further, an electromyography (EMG) study of case 8 established a dissociated injury of the Xth nerve with paresis of the soft palate and vocal fold, leaving the cricothyroid muscle intact. It has been suggested that a synchronized voltage in EMG studies is sometimes diagnostic of bulbar palsy (Sawaki et al., 1958; Hirose, 1984). Examinations by methods such as electroencephalography (EEG) (Bickerstaff, 1957) or cerebrospinal fuid (CSF) analysis (Arima et al., 1962) might be necessary in order to identify the etiological basis of the disorder.

Chronic Inflammatory Polyradiculoneuropathy

There are rare cases of idiopathic polyneuropathy that relapse or progress chronically (Ando et al., 1975; Arnason, 1975). They have been reported under the name of relapsing inflammatory polyradiculoneuropathy (Arnason, 1975), recurrent multiple cranial nerve palsy (Symonds, 1958), or polyneuritis cranialis (Toyokura, 1959). The clinical symptoms of this type of relapse do not differ essentially from those of the acute monophasic form of inflammatory polyradiculoneuropathy (Arnason, 1975). The etiology is unknown. An allergic reaction is suspected as in the case of the Guillain-Barré syndrome (Cody, 1946). In the present cases, there were five with relapsing or progressing palsy. Their clinical course closely resembles those of progressing multiple cranial neuropathy reported by Toyokura (1959). However, in the latter condition, the question whether a pure cranial nerve injury exists without peripheral nerve palsy is still controversial.

Chronic inflammatory polyradiculoneuropathy should be differentiated from degenerative diseases of the central nervous system, multiple sclerosis, sarcoidosis (Hirose, 1984), and chronic nonspecific inflammation of the skull base (Kamei, 1968).

CONCLUSION

Idiopathic associated laryngeal palsy is a rare condition in neurological symptomatology. It should be carefully differentiated from tumors, cerebrovascular disease, multiple sclerosis, sarcoidosis, and degenerative diseases of the nervous system. Even after such differentiation, a final diagnosis of "idiopathic" associated laryngeal palsy does not identify a single disease entity. Etiologically, the intranuclear, internuclear, or subnuclear injury resulting from an allergic reaction or viral infection can be postulated. In cases of acutely developing palsy with benign prognosis, three conditions have been suggested as possible causes: Guillain-Barré syndrome, direct invasion of herpes virus into the peripheral nervous system, or brainstem encephalitis. In almost one quarter of the present cases, the palsy was chronic or relapsing and resembled the clinical course of relapsing inflammatory polyradiculoneuropathy. However, in this rare condition, it is still controversial whether there exists a pure cranial nerve injury without other peripheral nerve palsy. In order to make a precise diagnosis from among the various possibilities outlined, it is important to describe accurately the clinical picture in the individual case, including the results of electrophysiological, serological, and CSF examinations.

The naming of classic eponymous syndromes applied to diseases affecting more than one cranial nerve is not practical for associated laryngeal palsy (Cody, 1946). The names suggest the location of injury only when a solitary lesion in the cranial nerve pathway disturbs a function peripheral to the injury. In "idiopathic" associated laryngeal palsy the clinical picture is not always the same: in brainstem encephalitis, combinations of cranial nerve injury develop according to the topography of the motoneuron pools in the brain stem; in viral infection, according to the relationship between individual peripheral nerves; and, in systemic reactions such as neuroallergy, the clinical manifestations are more random.

REFERENCES

Adour, K.K. (1976). Cranial polyneuritis and Bell's palsy. *Arch Otolaryng, 102,* 262–264.

Ando, K. et al. (1975). Idiopathic cranial polyneuritis. *Neurol Med JPN, 3,* 387–396.

Araki, S. (1974). *Neuropathy. Neurological medicine* (pp. 605–617). Tokyo: Kinpodo.

Arnason, B. (1975). Inflammatory polyradiculoneuropathies. In K. Dyck (Ed.), *Peripheral neuropathy* (pp. 1110–1148). Philadelphia: Sanders.

Arima, M. et al. (1962). The origin and the diagnosis of encephalitis in children. *Advances in Neurol Science JPN, 6,* 241–265.

Baringer, J.R. et al. (1975). Herpes virus infection of the peripheral nervous system. In Dyck (Ed.), *Peripheral Neuropathy* (pp. 1092–1103). Philadelphia: Saunders.

Bickerstaff, E.R. (1957). Brain-stem encephalitis. Further observation on a grave syndrome with benign prognosis. *Brit Med, 1,* 1384–1387.

Cody, C. C. (1946). Associated paralyses of the larynx. *Ann Otol Rhinol Laryngol, 55,* 549–561.

Djupesland, G., Degre, M., Stein, R., and Skrede, S. (1977). Acute peripheral facial palsy. Part of cranial polyneuropathy? *Arch Otolaryngol, 103,* 641–644.

Ellison, P.H., and Hanson, P.A. (1977). Herpes simplex: A possible cause of brain-stem encephalitis. *Pediatrics, 59,* 240–243.

Engstrom, H.E., and Wohlfart, G. (1949). Herpes zoster of the seventh, eighth, ninth and tenth cranial nerves. *Arch Neuro Psych, 62,* 638–652.

Font, J.H. (1952). The jugular foramen syndrome. *AMA Arch Otolaryngol, 56,* 134–141.

Hirayama, K. (1974). Clinical concept of the Guillain-Barré syndrome. *Neurolg Med JPN, 1,* 277–284.

Hirose, H. (1984). Associated laryngeal palsy. In H. Ishii (Ed.), *Recurrent nerva palsy* (pp. 184–196). Tokyo: Bunkodo.

Hunt, R. (1907). Herpetic inflammation of the geniculate ganglion: A new syndrome and its complications. *J Nerv & Ment Dis, 34,* 73–96.

Hunt, R. (1910). The symptom-complex of acute posterior poliomyelitis of the geniculate auditory glossopharyngeal and pneumogastric ganglia. *Arch Int Med, 5,* 631.

Igata, A. et al. (1974). The immunological aspect of the Guillain-Barré syndrome. *Neurol Med JPN, 1,* 297–305.

Ishii, H. et al. (1971). Inflammatory paralysis of the larynx. *J OtolaryngolJpn, 74,* 1562–1571.

Iwasa, H. et al. (1975). Localized encephalitis. A report of four cases. *Otolaryngology (Tokyo) 47,* 247–253.

Kamei, T. (1968). Six cases of associated laryngeal paralysis. *J Otolaryngol Jpn, 71,* 12–18.

Kawamura, K. et al. (1973). Clinical observation of patients with unilateral involvement of the last four cranial nerves. *Clin Neurol JPN, 13,* 196–202.

Konodo, K. et al. (1963). Eid idiopathische kranielle Polyneuritis. *Clin Neurol JPN, 3,* 167–173.

Lawn, A.M. (1966). The localization in the nucleus ambiguus of the rabbit of the cells of origin of motor nerve fibers in the glossopharyngeal nerve and various branches of the vagus nerve by means of retrograde degeneration. *J Comp Neur, 127,* 293–306.

Lewis, G.W. (1958). Zoster sine herpete. *Brit Med J, 2,* 418–421.

McCormick, D.P. (1972). Herpes-simplex virus as cause of Bell's palsy. *Lancet, 1,* 937–939.

Möller, F. (1956). Brain-stem encephalitis and epidemic vertigo. *Acta Psych Neurol Scand, 31,* 107–115.

Nozoe, I. et al. (1974). Polyneuritis cranialis -report of three cases -. *Otologia Fukuoka, 20,* 486–490.

Ogawa, A. et al. (1969). Clinical course of localized encephalitis in children. *J Pediatr Practice Jpn, 32,* 226–233.

Osler, L.D., Sidell, A.D. (1960). The Guillain-Barre syndrome. The need for exact diagnostic criteria. *New Engl J Med, 262,* 964–969.

Sato, I. et al. (1981). Idiopathic laryngeal nerve palsy and prevalence of influenza. *J Otolaryngol Jpn, 84,* 601–607.

Sawaki, S. et al. (1958). Disturbances of nucleus ambiguus with resulting manifestation of mixed paralysis of the larynx. *Otolaryngology (Tokyo) 30,* 736–738.

Shibata, H. et al. (1975). A case of idiopathic acute cranial polyneuritis. *Med J Minami-Osaka Hosp, 23,* 53–56.

Sobue, I. (1974). Clinical features and variants of the Guillain-Barré syndrome. *Neurol Med JPN, 1,* 321–328.

Symonds, C. (1958). Recurrent multiple cranial nerve palsies. *J Neurol Neurosurg Psychiat, 21,* 95.

Toyokura, Y. (1959). Cranial polyneuritis: Report of a case. *Int Med JPN, 3,* 231–238.

Vernet, M. (1918). The classification of the syndromes of associated laryngeal palsy. *J Laryngol Rhinol Otol, 33,* 354–365.

Wells, C.E.C. (1971). Neurological complications of so-called "influenza"; A winter study in southeast Wales. *Brit Med J, 13,* 369–373.

Wiederholt, W.C. et al. (1964). The Landry-Guillain-Barré-Strohl syndrome or polyradiculoneuropathy. Historical review, report on 97 patients and present concept. *Mayo Clin Proc, 39,* 427.

Wyke, B.D., and Kirchner, J.A. (1976). Neurology of the larynx. In R. Hinchcliffe (Ed.), *Scientific foundations of otolaryngology* (pp. 546–574). London: Hinemann.

Yoshida, Y. et al. (1982). Laryngeal motoneurons of cats. *J Otolaryng Jpn, 85,* 455–463.

CHAPTER 22

Laryngeal Behavior in Patients with Disorders of the Central Nervous System

Hajime HIROSE
and Yutaka JOSHITA

Dysarthric speech is often a cardinal symptom of disorders of the central nervous system. The pattern of dysarthrias differs depending on the type of disease and on the severity of the pathology, but, in most cases, certain aspects of both articulation and prosody are affected to varying degrees (Darley, Aronson, and Brown, 1975).

As for abnormalities in prosody, a breakdown in the temporal pattern of speech generally dominates, but phonatory disturbances related to the control of vocal pitch and intensity may occur as well. Further, an abnormal quality of the voice often accompanies dysarthric speech, as, for example, in parkinsonism (Logemann, Boshes, and Fisher, 1973). Amyotrophic lateral sclerosis (ALS) or pseudo-bulbar palsy (PBP) may produce a monotonous, choked, or strained voice. The larynx, then, is often a victim of these disorders.

Participation of the larynx in articulatory adjustments has been well documented. In particular, the adduction-abduction control of the vocal folds plays a principal role in the voiced-voiceless distinction for consonant production (Hirose and Sawashima, 1981). Thus, the analysis of laryngeal dynamics related to the articulatory and phonatory functions in dysarthric subjects is an important element in the clinical evaluation of dysarthrias.

This paper will describe some of the clinical features of different types of dysarthria with respect to laryngeal dynamics in voice and speech production. Each dysarthric subject underwent otolaryngological and phoniatric examinations at the time of speech evaluation. In selected cases, laryngeal maneuvers during speech production were analyzed using photoglottography (PGG), electromyography (EMG), or both.

PGG AND EMG PROCEDURES

Figure 22-1 shows a block diagram of the PGG recordings. A fiberscope was inserted through a nostril of each subject. The fiberscope was attached to a video camera and, while the glottal maneuvers were displayed on a monitor screen, the illumination modulated by the glottal gestures was sensed by a phototransistor attached to the anterior neck at the level of the trachea. The signals were recorded on a PCM data recorder.

In the PGG data recording sessions, subjects were required to repeat the Japanese monosyllables /se/ and /he/ as quickly and as regularly as possible. In addition, different types of meaningful Japanese words embedded in a carrier phrase were also recorded.

EMG signals were recorded from the thyroarytenoid muscle during phonation and respiration using a conventional bipolar needle electrode. In selected cases, other laryngeal and tongue muscles were also examined.

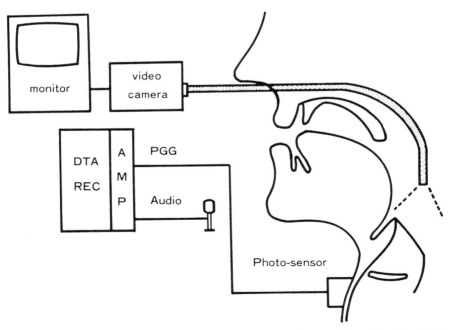

Figure 22-1. *Block diagram of the photoglottography (PGG) procedure with video-image monitoring.*

RESULTS AND COMMENTS

Normal Subject

PGG patterns of normal subjects were examined and used as controls before analyzing the abnormal patterns of laryngeal behavior in dysarthric cases with central nervous system disorders.

Figure 22-2 shows a PGG record obtained from a normal subject during repetition of the monosyllable /se/. The upward shift of the curve indicates the glottal opening gesture. It is apparent that the glottis opened and closed regularly during rhythmic repetition of the monosyllable, which consisted of a voiceless consonant and a vowel. The degree of glottal opening represented by the height of the upward shift appears to be consistent.

Figure 22-3 shows another photoglottogram obtained from the same normal subject during repetition of the monosyllable /he/. Glottal opening and closing was maintained at a regular rhythm, although the degree of glottal opening gradually decreased toward the end of the series of repetitions.

Amyotrophic Lateral Sclerosis (ALS)

PGG analysis was made for two ALS patients. In both patients, the range of vocal fold movements for the adduction and abduction gesture was within normal limits. However, both patients had some difficulty in the syllable repetition task, and there was a tendency for subjects to adduct the false fold during phonation. This resulted in very tight glottal closure, which produced a strained or choked vocal quality.

A glottogram obtained from one of the ALS cases during repetition of the monosyllable /he/ is shown

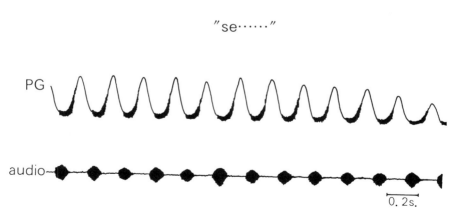

Figure 22-2. *Photoglottogram (PG) and speech envelope (audio) obtained from a normal subject in repetitions of the monosyllable /se/ displayed as time functions.*

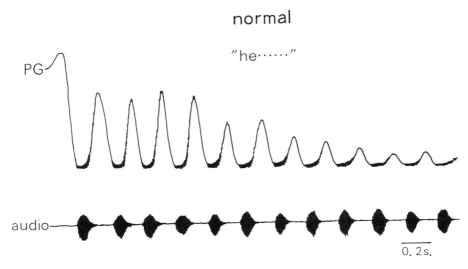

normal

"he······"

PG

audio

0. 2s.

Figure 22-3. *PG obtained from a normal subject in repetitions of the monosyllable /he/.*

in Figure 22-4. Compared to the normal pattern, repetitive gestures of the glottis quickly became irregular. The glottal opening became smaller, and the pattern of the repetitive glottal gestures became irregular. The voiceless /h/ appeared to be replaced by a voiced /h/. The fifth repetition was preceded by an interval of glottal opening, associated with an abrupt intake of air, followed by a choking gesture with an outbreak of coughing, as shown by the arrow in the figure. The choking gesture seems to have resulted from a tight reflex glottic closure associated with increasing spasticity.

The glottal gestures of choking followed by an outbreak of coughing can also be seen in Figure 22-5A, which shows the same ALS subject's utterance of the Japanese sentence "sore o kisse to yuu" (We call that kisse). The choking occurred at the end of the carrier portion of "sero o," and the subsequent outbreak of coughing is indicated by an arrow. In contrast to the normal pattern (Figure 22-5B), the ALS subject did not produce a devoicing of /i/ between /k/ and /s/ in the test word.

In the EMG examination, there was a decrease in the neuromuscular unit (NMU) discharges associated with high amplitude voltage units often appearing synchronously in both the laryngeal and tongue muscles, suggesting multiple involvement of secondary neurons in the cranial nerve region.

Parkinsonism

It has often been noted that parkinsonian subjects tend automatically to repeat the same articulatory gesture, or to "stutter," during speech. Figure 22-6 shows the

ALS

"he······"

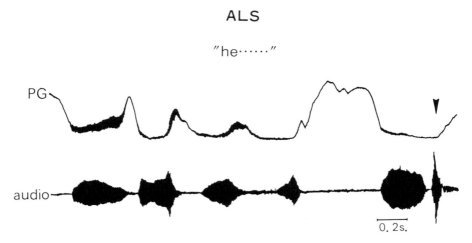

Figure 22-4. *PG obtained from subject with ALS in repetitions of the monosyllable /he/.*

glottogram of a parkinsonian sub-ject during production of the test word /kisse/ embedded in the car-rier "sore o ____ to yuu." The sub-ject seems to repeat the articula-tory gesture for producing /k/, but the laryngeal gesture appears to be nearly closed. This pattern is quite similar to that observed in a case of developmental stuttering (Yoshioka and Lofqvist, 1981).

Phoniatric studies on parkinson-ian subjects have often revealed that parkinsonian patients, as a group, speak at significantly higher pitch levels and with signifi-cantly less pitch variability than normal control subjects (Canter, 1965). In our study of 34 cases of parkinsonism (24 male and 10 female subjects), only 11 out of the 24 male subjects had a higher speaking pitch, whereas among the female subjects, none showed a higher speaking pitch. However, 8 out of the 10 female subjects had a lower speaking pitch than the normal controls. Thus, a sex-

related difference must be taken into consideration before making a general description of pitch lev-els in parkinsonian subjects. Vocal tremor and a breathy character of voice are often observed.

It has been reported that parkin-sonian subjects may develop laryngeal paralysis in the course of the disease (Plasse and Lieber-man, 1981). In these reports, how-ever, the diagnosis of laryngeal paralysis has been made simply by observation under convention-al laryngoscopy. Although parkin-sonian subjects often present a very weak, breathy voice associat-ed with limited movements of the vocal folds, a definite diagnosis of paralysis can be made only by electromyography.

Figure 22-7 shows the EMG pat-terns for the thyroarytenoid ob-tained from a parkinsonian patient who showed very limited vocal fold movements under indirect laryn-goscopy. The EMGs were record-ed during a series of alternating in-

A

ALS

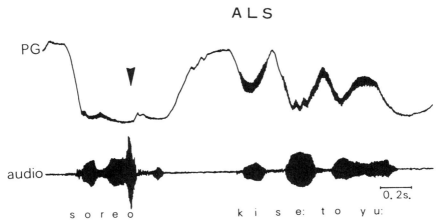

B

normal

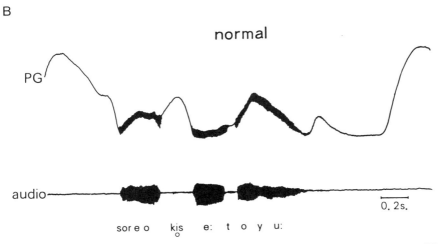

Figure 22-5. *PG obtained from a subject with ALS (A) and a normal subject (B) in production of the Japanese test utterence "sore o kisse to yuu."*

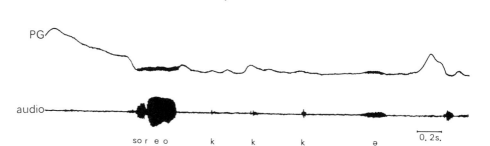

Figure 22-6. *PG obtained from a subject with parkinsonism in production of the test utterence "sore o kisse to yuu."*

spiration and phonation. It appears that the number of NMU discharges during phonation, or during the concomitant vocal fold adduction, is not reduced, nor are there any pathological discharge patterns, such as polyphasic or high amplitude voltages. On the other hand, persistent firing can be seen even during the period of inspiration, in which thyroarytenoid activity is normally suppressed . The findings in this case indicate that there is no neurogenic paralysis, but that there is a loss of the reciprocal suppression of the thyroarytenoid during inspiration.

Hypokinetic patterns in parkinsonism in terms of a reduction in the range of movements can be related to deterioration in the reciprocal adjustment of the antagonistic muscles. The limitation of vocal fold movements in this case is probably an example of this type of disorder. The EMG pattern of persistent discharges in the thyroarytenoid muscle must be taken as physiological evidence of parkinsonian rigidity as described by Leanderson, Meyerson, and

Persson (1972). These investigators found persistent EMG discharges in functionally antagonistic pairs of facial muscles of parkinsonian subjects.

Although EMG signals were not recorded from the functionally antagonistic muscle, the posterior cricoarytenoid (PCA) in this case, it seems probable that the apparent limitation of vocal fold mobility was due to the rigidity of the laryngeal muscles caused by parkinsonism. Thus, we hold the view that the apparent limitation of vocal fold movements in parkinsonian patients should not be regarded as vocal fold paralysis.

Shy-Drager Syndrome

The Shy-Drager syndrome was first reported as a clinical entity resulting from degenerative disease and manifested by orthostatic hypotension. Recent studies suggest that the syndrome is due to multiple system atrophy of the autonomic nervous system, particularly in the central region. Clinically, laryngeal stridor has been

Parkinsonism   EH 51f

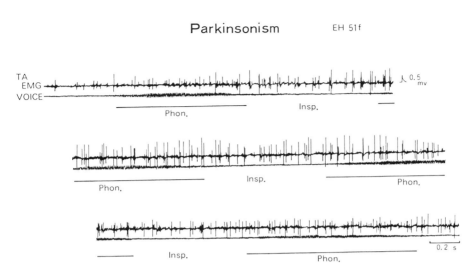

Figure 22-7. *EMG patterns for the thyroarytenoid (TA) obtained from a subject with parkinsonism in a series of alternating phonation and inspiration.*

observed to be an important symptom of the Shy-Drager syndrome. Laryngeal examination often reveals limitation of vocal fold abduction associated with inspiratory stridor. This is usually worse during sleep and can produce periodic nocturnal apnea. Difficulty in swallowing is another important feature of the syndrome, and pooling of saliva in the pyriform sinus is frequently observed on laryngeal examination.

Tomonaga (1985) reported neurogenic atrophy in the PCA of a 58-year-old female subject with Shy-Drager syndrome studied at autopsy, whereas there was no evidence of degenerative change in the nucleus ambiguus. This result is comparable to the case reported by Bannister, Gibson, Michaels, and Oppenheimer (1981), and suggests that the origin of the neurogenic atrophy of the PCA was situated at a more peripheral level.

ACKNOWLEDGMENT

The authors wish to express their appreciation to the staff of the Research Institute of Logopedics and Phoniatrics and Department of Neurology (Chairman: Prof. T. Mannen), Faculty of Medicine, University of Tokyo, and the Department of Neurology (Chairman: Prof. M. Yoshida), Jichi Medical School. This study was supported in part by the Grant-in-Aid for Scientific Research from the Ministry of Education of the Japanese Government.

REFERENCES

Bannister, R., Gibson, W., Michaels, L., and Oppenheimer, D.R. (1981). Laryngeal abductor paralysis in multiple system atrophy. A report on three necropsied cases, with observations on the laryngeal muscles and the nuclei ambiguui. *Brain, 104,* 351–368.

Canter, G.J. (1965). Speech characteristics of patients with Parkinson's disease: II. Physiological support of speech. *Jour Speech Hear Dis, 30,* 44–49.

Darley, F.L., Aronson, A.E., and Brown, J.R. (1975). *Motor speech disorders.* Philadelphia: Saunders.

Hirose, H., and Sawashima, M. (1981). Functions of the laryngeal muscles in speech. In K.N. Stevens and M. Hirano (Eds.), *Vocal fold physiology* (pp. 137–154). Tokyo: University of Tokyo Press.

Leanderson, R., Meyerson, B.A., and Persson, A. (1972). Lip muscle function in parkinsonian dysarthria. *Acta Otolaryngol, 74,* 354–357.

Logemann, J., Boshes, B., and Fisher, H. (1973). The steps in the degeneration of speech and voice in Parkinson's disease. In G. Siegfried (Ed.), *Parkinson diseases Vol. 2* (pp. 101–112). Bern: Hans Huber.

Plasse, H.M., and Lieberman, A.N. (1981). Bilateral vocal cord paralysis in Parkinson's disease. *Arch Otolaryngol, 107,* 252–253.

Tomonaga, M. (1985). Pathology of Shy-Drager syndrome - With special reference to the autonomic nervous system -. *Brain and Nerve, 37,* 687–689.

Yoshioka, H., and Lofqvist, A. (1981). Laryngeal involvement in stuttering — A glottographic observation using a reaction time paradigm -. *Folia Phoniat. 33,* 348–357.

AUTHOR INDEX

SUBJECT INDEX